STOP CANCER WITH PHYTOTHERAPY

With 100+ anti-cancer recipes

Benjamin Lau, MD, PhD
and
Esther Lau, MS, RD

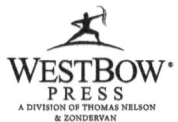

WESTBOW®
PRESS
A DIVISION OF THOMAS NELSON
& ZONDERVAN

WestBow Press books may be ordered through booksellers or by contacting:

WestBow Press
A Division of Thomas Nelson & Zondervan
1663 Liberty Drive
Bloomington, IN 47403
www.westbowpress.com
1 (866) 928-1240

ISBN: 978-1-4908-4810-5 (sc)
ISBN: 978-1-4908-4812-9 (hc)
ISBN: 978-1-4908-4811-2 (e)

Library of Congress Control Number: 2014914849

Printed in the United States of America.

WestBow Press rev. date: 09/05/2014

DEDICATED
TO
ANNA H. WANG, RN

This book is dedicated to Esther's 103-year-old mother whose zest for life and whose avant-garde foresight led her to nutritional and health practices which are only now being confirmed by science. For half a century, she served freshly extracted juices to the residents of her 50-bed nursing home in Illinois, and even today she still drinks her two cups of carrot juice every morning. Amazingly, her thinning white hair is now being replaced by a thick new growth of black hair! Always enjoying learning, she learned to crochet shortly before her 100th birthday – an activity she enjoys daily. A recent physical exam revealed a remarkably healthy woman with all the indices of an individual half her age. And it is to this living monument of sound nutritional and health practices that we lovingly dedicate this book.

"This is a great book for you.
It is very true.
It tells you how to get well,
And make you happy and swell!"

Unedited poem by Kyra Kaya, 8-year-old
great granddaughter of Anna H. Wang

CONTENTS

Acknowledgments

For a period of more than three decades, I have had the privilege of working with a good number of graduate students, postdoctoral fellows, and colleagues whose findings are included in this book. I wish to acknowledge the following individuals: Moses Adetumbi, PhD, George Javor, PhD, Padma Tadi-Uppala, PhD, Jeff Tosk, PhD, Robert Teel, PhD, Lin Li, MD, PhD, Takeshi Yamasaki, DVM, Christopher Marsh, MD, James Woolley, MD, Daila Gridley, PhD, Brian Wong, PhD, Clifford Herrmann, PhD, Jian Qian, MD, Yu Wang, MD, Chok Wan, MD, PhD, Roger Hadley, MD, Gary Barker. MD, Robert Torrey, MD, Dick Koobs, MD, PhD, Herbert Ruckle, MD, Jerry Rittenhouse, MD, Paul Lui, MD, Tomi Botolazzo, MD, Robert Myers, MD, James Slater, MD, Douglas Wong, MD, Amber Buz'Zard, PhD, Nagatoshi Ide, PhD, William Chu, PhD, Ted Masek, MD, Ernest Ngo, MD, Judy Johnson, MS, Erben Bayeta, MS, Vandana Shah, MS, Peck Ong, MD, James Kettering, PhD, Charles Winter, PhD. Heidi Ngo, MD, and Becky Wang, MD.

I wish to acknowledge the financial support for my research from the Chan Shun Research Fund for AIDS and Cancer (Chan Shun International Foundation, Burlingame, California).

My sister-in-law Ruth Liu, EdD, has spent many hours to read and polish up the book manuscript, for which we are most grateful. Finally, I want to thank our publisher for doing a superb job in making this book available to the public.

A SYNOPSIS

We propose a new paradigm to stop cancer, using a novel therapy called phytotherapy or plant-based nutrition:

Phytotherapy is the most advanced immunotherapy based on our own research.

Phytotherapy is the safest chemotherapy as it has no adverse side effects, again based on our own research.

Phytotherapy is a non-invasive surgery. It can eliminate cancer without the scalpel, based on our own research and clinical observation.

This book tells you how to Stop Cancer. You may be told that there is no other way than through chemotherapy, radiation and surgery. But we offer for the first time phytotherapy's triple action capable of stopping a deadly killer disease taking more than 600,000 lives every year in the United States.

Phytotherapy is *immunotherapy*. A plant-based diet provides thousands of phytonutrients that feeds the immune cells and enhances their functions. Our own research clearly demonstrates that the immune system is the body's best and only bullet-proof defense against cancer.

Phytotherapy is *chemotherapy* without the adverse side effects. Phytochemicals (plant chemicals) have been shown to selectively destroy cancer cells while non-toxic to normal cells. Most of the current patented chemotherapeutic drugs destroy both the cancerous along with the healthy cells – that is, they kill and weaken every cell indiscriminately. However, phytochemicals can provide dual functions – selectively killing only cancer cells while supplying nutrients to enrich normal cells.

Phytotherapy is a *non-surgical surgery*. In our animal studies and clinical observations, plant chemicals have been shown to cause cancer/tumor to fall off from the body naturally without a scalpel.

We are living in a most momentous time, unparalleled in human history. We are winning the war on cancer through the use of a plant-based diet. Phytotherapy has finally emerged as the long-waited breakthrough. Its significance impacts many lives saved, relationships restored, and future dreams realized.

Indeed we are a fortuitous generation. We can no longer ignore the importance of nutrition and lifestyles in fighting cancer. This is precisely what propels us with an urgent message that *what we eat and how we live* can prevent, arrest, and reverse cancer. Our only desire is to share with you what we have learned so that every man, woman and child can control his/her own destiny living cancer-free.

Simple Solutions in a Nutshell

If you have cancer or someone you know of has cancer, here are some brief guidelines you may wish to incorporate immediately:

1. Stop eating all animal products and processed foods as these promote cancer growth.
2. Eat an unprocessed plant-based diet with thousands of phytochemicals that destroy cancer cells and strengthen immune cells.
3. Go to sleep every night before 10 pm.
4. If the tumor is small, sit tight. If the tumor is large, you may opt to have it surgically removed.
5. If it is too difficult for you to do it on your own, you may consider spending some time to learn how to change your diet and lifestyle habits in a wellness center (see appendix).

Take time to consider all your options. Do not rush into any hasty decisions. A cancer diagnosis can be an impetus towards healthier living in which one can experience the best years yet to come!

PREFACE

Are we close to finding a cure for cancer?

The number of cancer survivors has increased since the 1970s when President Nixon signed the National Cancer Act. Yet cancer remains a complex disease too canny to be eradicated anytime soon.

Unless and until we make some changes!

Many years ago, I (Esther) recall in my mother's kitchen often hearing that familiar hum of the juicer spewing out carrot and other vegetable juice. Next would be the splish-splash sound of the fresh juices filling the Mason jars. Then armed with the precious cargo, my mother would faithfully begin her round of deliveries to those facing the ravages of cancer, some of whom were reeling with the dreaded verdict of their doctors: "There's nothing more we can do."

My mother's care and compassion fueled her loving service to others, as she daily drove across town often combating the severe Illinois winters. Along with fresh juices she graciously extended comfort to the despondent and hope to the hopeless.

One such recipient was a massage therapist diagnosed with advanced stage of breast cancer who resigned herself to impending death. But to the utter amazement of family and friends, rather than closing down her life, she re-opened her massage business and enjoyed many happy, productive years far beyond her doctor's prediction.

Being young, foolish, and skeptical at that time, I would defiantly challenge my mother with, "Mom, I'm getting my master's degree from UC Berkeley, and I know there's no such magic in carrot or any other vegetable juice!" But undaunted, she nevertheless presented us our wedding gift – a heavy duty juicer. This I promptly stored unopened in my bottom kitchen cabinet, never to be touched until....

"Your son has lymphoma!"

Those chilling words from the surgeon struck a terror in my heart! Just that morning 13-year-old Danny had undergone an elective surgery to remove a nodule under his chin — merely for cosmetic reasons. My husband Ben had assured me that the nodule was due to infectious mononucleosis from a few months ago, nothing serious.

But the surgeon's words shocked me back to reality: "I have arranged for him to start chemo tomorrow." With that, he swiveled around and marched out of the room.

Wait, wait, what did he say? Lymphoma? Chemo? Tomorrow?

My mind whirled, my heart pounded. I had to sit down, so I dashed down the hall to the empty waiting room, collapsing on the couch.

"O, God. No! No, please." A torrent of tears streamed down my face. "Lord, don't you remember? This is *the* child that we had prayed for, for six years," I sobbed.

How cruel life seemed! I had just finished reading a heart wrenching story about a mother losing her teenage son to cancer. In fact, few years ago, I had tried to comfort this very mother shortly after her tragic loss.

"Please don't take *my* son too. Can You *hear* me???" I couldn't breathe. I felt faint....

Of all days, Ben was in Los Angeles, two hours away, for a meeting. What should I do? What *could* I do?

Finally, I stood to my feet. With firm resolve, I uttered an audible "No! No chemo tomorrow." I need time....

After enduring two interminably long hours, I heard Ben bounce jovially into the hospital room with his usual boisterous "Hah-lo!" But, one glance at my face froze his smile as I quickly relayed the doctor's verdict.

"No, it can't be! It must be a wrong diagnosis!" With that, he headed to the nurses' station where he read the pathology report and then consulted his pathology professor and a senior resident. After a few more phone calls, he bounded back into our son's room and asked, "Ready to go home, Son?"

With cautious optimism, I breathed a sigh of relief. At least, no chemo tomorrow!

Our first brush with cancer, fortunately, turned out well. Lymphoma was a misdiagnosis, as pathology reports from other labs in Southern California concurred with Ben. But what about the millions of people who have not been so fortunate?

Three decades have passed. Cancer rages on!

INTRODUCTION

"You have cancer...." Three chilling words. Three cruel words. Yet with unleashed power, they deliver a devastating blow, taking more than 600,000 lives every year in the United States alone. The incidence of cancer is escalating at an alarming rate! Something must be done.

Over 1.6 million new cases of cancer are being diagnosed annually in the U.S. Furthermore, despite advances in modern technology and treatment, over a half-million people die each year from this dreaded disease.[1] In fact, the annual death rate from cancers is roughly one-third of the number of new cases diagnosed. But for those suffering from stomach and colon cancers, the mortality rate stands even higher, at 50 percent; and for those with liver, pancreas and lung cancers, it may even be over 80 percent!

"The Cancer Project" of the PCRM (Physicians Committee for Responsible Medicine) estimates that one out of every two men and one out of every three women in the U.S. are at risk for cancer. The most common type for men is prostate cancer, while breast cancer is the most common type in women.[2] Breast cancer has increased significantly in the past 50 years, from 62,000 new cases in 1960 to over 200,000 in 2010 – more than a three-fold increase![3] Other types of cancer also show a steady annual increase. Why is there such an increase? I will tell you why in later chapters. Once you know the causes, you are in a better position to understand how to prevent and maybe even reverse the cancer.

Not only is the problem exploding exponentially here in the U.S., but globally, cancer is also growing at an alarming pace. An estimated 7.6 million people died of cancer in 2005 and 84 million people will die in the next 10 years if action is not taken.[4] The World Health Organization warns that new cancer cases worldwide are predicated to jump from 14 million in 2012 to 22 million every year within the next two decades.[5,6] By the year 2020, approximately 15 million new cases will be diagnosed, and 12 million cancer patients will die.[7]

Such statistics are troubling at multiple levels, one of which is the effect upon the current health care crisis, an enormous challenge facing our country. Health costs have escalated to the point of no return, unless drastic changes are made.

In 2010, taxpayers paid nearly $2.6 trillion for healthcare services, a tenfold jump from 1980.[8] Over 17% of the country's GDP (gross domestic product) is spent on health care – much more than any other nation. Yet despite the enormous spending, how tragic that our country has lower life expectancy rates and higher heart disease, and cancer rates than other civilized nations.[9]

Now with the health care crisis in this country fueled by the escalation of cost not only in dollars, but also in non-productivity, disability, and death – something has to be done. The obvious solution is a paradigm shift that is long overdue. Rather than incurring the exorbitant costs (financial, physical, emotional) of treating a disease after the fact, why not prevent it in the first place?

Neal Barnard, MD, president of Physicians Committee for Responsible Medicine (PCRM), recently stated that "80 percent of cancers are influenced by controllable circumstances, including diet." He further admonished, "The link between diet and cancer is too big to be ignored and it is more critical than ever that you and your loved ones have the resources available to learn how your diet can play a key role in the prevention of cancer. And, if cancer is diagnosed, that the foods you eat can increase your chances for survival."[10] In this book I'll elaborate in more details these points made by Dr. Barnard.

When I visited China 30 years ago, China was one of those few countries in the world with relatively low incidence of cancer. Today, there is a 30-fold increase in breast cancer and colon cancer compared with 30 years ago. Why is there such a significant increase? I will tell you a little later. Meanwhile, I would like for you to think of some of the things that may be responsible for such increase—think about what are differences today in China compared with 30 or 40 years ago.

Who doesn't long for a healthy life, filled with meaning, joy, and exuberance, shared with those we love? Is there anything we can do to increase our chances for this kind of life? Is there anything we can do to decrease our chances for illness?

The answer is yes. While much in our lives is not in our control, there is still much that *is* in our control, and it is in these arenas where we can learn to make wise choices that can not only decrease our chances of getting cancer (and a host of other diseases) but can also increase our chances for vibrant health. In this book we want to emphasize that *diet and lifestyle modification can help to prevent, arrest, and reverse cancer!*

According to Dr. Richard H. Carmona, Surgeon General of the United States (2002-2006), 75% of the expenditure for health care is spent on diseases that are totally preventable. A staggering 40% of all cancer deaths is preventable.[4] Simple lifestyle changes could decrease cancer risk by 38% for breast cancer, 45% for colon cancer, and 47% for stomach cancer.[11] Dr. Carmona suggests that we ought to pay people for staying healthy.[12]

We believe that cancer is predominantly a lifestyle disease – the way we eat and how we live. Eighty to 90 percent of all cancers are linked to our poor dietary practices, smoking, and exposure to environmental toxins. Today an ever-increasing body of research supports the role of lifestyle in health and disease, but the pioneering researchers faced severe opposition to their published data.

In the 1980s, the lone voice of Dr. Dean Ornish, contrary to then-current medical wisdom, declared that heart diseases can be reversed with diet and lifestyle modifications.[13] Understandably, such a claim was not well received by the medical community or the lay public.

Then another trailblazer, surgeon Dr. Caldwell B. Esselstyn, from the renowned Cleveland Clinic, found similar results through his research – that a strict plant-based diet, regardless of amount of exercise, could reverse coronary heart disease.[14]

In recent decades, the works of Dr. Neal Barnard and others found that diabetes can also be reversed with a plant-based diet and proper lifestyle.[15]

Thus begs the question: If heart diseases and diabetes can be reversed, can cancer also be reversed through diet and lifestyle? The answer is yes. Exciting news indeed!

In his landmark nutrition research, Dr. T. Colin Campbell clearly demonstrated that certain foods can turn cancer "on" and "off."[16] In other words, each individual can potentially influence his or her destiny in the prevention and reversal of cancer!

Interestingly, Dr. John McDougall, another pioneer in nutrition research and practice for more than four decades promoted a plant-based diet along with healthy lifestyle for the prevention and treatment of diseases. And pinpointing cancer, Dr. McDougall states that "Most knowledgeable people now believe that our rich American diet is an important factor in causing cancers of the breast, colon, prostate, and other organs."[17]

Thus, substantiated by compelling scientific data, we now know that just as heart disease and diabetes can be reversed through diet and lifestyle, cancer too can be prevented, arrested, and reversed by diet and lifestyle modification.

One of the greatest single reasons for the devastating cancer toll is ignorance – what causes cancer, how to prevent it, and how to treat it. Knowledge is power, and with knowledge, you can make informed choices. And that is the purpose of this book – to empower you to actively participate in your own health and wellness and to provide you with life-enhancing tools. Because the human body has amazing healing ability, we propose a total program that encompasses the physical, mental, and spiritual components to enable the body to heal itself.

The remainder of this book focuses on:

➢ The basic and clinical cancer research conducted by the author as well as by other reputable researchers; plus observational research data collected around the world.
➢ The role of the immune system in cancer prevention and recovery.
➢ Factors that contribute to cancer;
➢ The prevention and reversal of cancer through the 3-R Diet and the Newstart® lifestyle program.

The underlying message of this book is that regardless of one's choice of treatment (surgery, chemotherapy, radiation, a combination of treatments or no treatment), most important of all is to:

- ✓ **Stop doing the things that make you sick.**
- ✓ **Start doing the things that will make you well.**

CHAPTER 1

WHY THIS BOOK?

There must be a logical answer on how to stop cancer. Allow me to say right here in the beginning that *phytotherapy* is the answer. In this book we will share with you our own laboratory research along with observational studies for supporting this thesis.

We know that all of us may have a few cancer cells in our bodies at any given time. But not everyone develops cancer. Why? Because we are each endowed with an incredibly amazing powerful defense mechanism called the immune system. Our immune function, particularly the type called the *natural immunity* (described in Chapter 5), has the capability of destroying cancer cells upon contact. That is, if our immune system remains strong.

Early in my research career using animal models, I studied surgery, chemotherapy, radiation, immunotherapy, and nutritional therapy for treating cancer.[1,2,3] I also used crude extracts of garlic, several Chinese medicinal herbs, and other phytochemicals (plant chemicals). I discovered that all the different modalities were effective in controlling cancer in the experimental animals. However, I found that phytochemicals turned out to be most effective. Let me explain.

We know that quite a number of chemotherapeutic agents used for treating cancer were originally derived from plants. When they are purified, most chemotherapeutic agents carry serious side effects. When I used the crude extracts from plants, I discovered that they were as effective as the chemotherapeutic agents in killing cancer cells. But with one notable difference: the crude extracts showed little or no side effects while patented chemotherapeutic drugs were quite toxic to the animals! That was an important knowledge I gained in my early research career.

There are three well-known causes for cancer: chemical carcinogens, radiation, and microorganisms, particularly viruses. All of them can enter into our normal cells and cause their DNA to mutate or change into cancer-prone cells. However, small numbers of cancer-prone cells are readily destroyed by our immune cells, such as macrophages and natural killer cells both of which are members of the natural immunity my associates and I studied a great deal in our laboratory. That is good because our immune cells are powerful and vigilant in protecting our bodies from invaders!

Cancer development goes through three stages: initiation, promotion, and progression:

1. Initiation: In this stage, an agent enters a normal cell, gets into its nucleus and changes its DNA, and turns this cell into a cancer-prone cell. Rather than following the normal growth pattern, it goes berserk as it continues to produce more cancer-prone cells, finally growing a small tumor or a colony onsite.
2. Promotion: At this juncture, the small colony/tumor feeds on special nutrients (promoter food) that make it grow and extend to the adjacent area.
3. Progression: Finally, the tumor grows wild and spreads to distant areas.

Immune cells can easily rid the cancer-prone cells in the initiation stage but may not be so easily in promotion and progression stages because of the *blindfolding* and *cover-up* tactics employed by cancer cells. But do not get disheartened. Let me hasten to tell you that our numerous studies have now shown that phytochemicals can actually abolish all three stages of cancer development, meaning they can stop initiation, promotion, and progression, detailed in Chapter 2.

What is blindfolding? It's a war-like tactic, an escape mechanism, used by cancer cells to protect themselves from the attacks of the approaching immune cells. How do the cancer cells blindfold our immune cells, such as natural killer cells and macrophages? They spray them with soluble factors (antigens). And exactly what constitute these soluble factors? You can probably guess. The cancer cells use their own excreta!

The excreta-like soluble factors act like handkerchiefs that can actually blindfold the immune cells. In the meantime, the blinded immune cells become disillusioned into thinking that they have already done a good job of destroying the cancer cells. In other words, our immune cells are blinded and fooled; in reality, they fail to destroy the cancer cells. But don't get discouraged—it's really not that bad. As I mentioned a minute ago, our numerous studies have shown that feeding the immune cells with phytochemicals can instantly enable them to remove the handkerchiefs and restore them to kill cancer cells again![4,5]

What is the cover-up? This is another escape mechanism used by cancer cells to protect themselves by covering their cell surfaces with a protein coating. Thus our immune cells cannot recognize the cancer cells with their cover-up, or new coat. What constitutes this cover-up coating? It is animal protein from our diet. How so?

Normally the protein coating on the cancer cell surfaces can be easily destroyed or digested by our body's pancreatic enzymes (trypsin and chymotrypsin). However, when animal protein is consumed, the enzymes are used up to digest animal protein in the diet so that there will not be enough enzymes available to digest the protein coating on the surfaces of the cancer cells. That is why eating animal foods can actually protect cancer and fend off our immune helpers. When we stop animal protein consumption, there will be adequate supply of trypsin and chymotrypsin to digest the protein coating on the cancer cells. Then our immune cells will recognize the cancer cells because they are without their camouflaged coats. Interestingly, eating plant protein does not consume our pancreatic enzymes trypsin and chymotrypsin. Plant protein does not contribute to cancer cover-up. Not only that, our studies show phytochemicals greatly maximize the immune function to destroy cancer cells.[6] Furthermore, phytochemicals are selectively toxic to cancer cells while nourishing to normal healthy cells (discussed in Chapters 3 and 7). This is exciting!

In recent years we have been hearing a lot about *angiogenesis* or new blood vessel development, an important process in cancer progression or metastasis. In the early 1970s, scientists discovered that cancer cells can secrete growth factors that stimulate angiogenesis with growth of new blood vessels.[7] Cancer cells can thus spread to distant sites via the new blood vessels they help to create. It's like building their bridge. In this past decade, scientists have been busy in researching new drugs to halt the angiogenesis process so as to stop cancer progression. However, while waiting for the new drugs to be developed, nutritionists have already discovered that many fruits and vegetables have anti-angiogenic property.[8] The list includes common food items such as apples, artichokes, different kinds of berries, broccoli, cabbage, cauliflower, garlic, kale, lemons, oranges, tomatoes, and many others. So eating these foods can stop cancer cells from making new blood vessels. Again, this shows phytochemicals are indeed powerful!

For over three decades our own laboratory studies have shown that phytochemicals or nutritional therapy can enhance all our immune cell functions (macrophages, natural killer cells and T lymphocytes) to potentiate their ability to destroy cancer cells. In recent years, we have seen that nutritional therapy is, indeed, most powerful in stopping cancer.

Our own research, both observational and clinical studies all confirm that phyto- or nutritional therapy can effectively stop cancer. In this book, you will read about research from other scientists supporting this thesis as well. In the second part of the book we will give you instructions on how to use phytotherapy along with lifestyle changes to stop cancer.

Why this book? It is written with you in mind. It is our desire to share what we have learned with you, our fellow travelers, on this journey to stop cancer by doing the following:

1. Stop doing things that have brought on cancer;
2. Start doing things that strengthen your immune system to stop cancer once and for all.

How do we go about doing these things? You will find the details in the second part of this book.

CHAPTER 2

BEGINNINGS OF
CANCER RESEARCH

After receiving my PhD from the University of Kentucky with an emphasis in immunology and medical microbiology, I returned to Hinsdale, Illinois, a suburban town near Chicago, to resume my responsibility as a medical microbiologist and director of a new research laboratory in a community hospital. Prior to my graduate study, I was employed as a microbiologist in this same hospital. I had only stayed in Hinsdale for a little over two years when I accepted a teaching and research position as an assistant professor at Loma Linda University Medical School in Southern California.

My work in the medical school was full of excitement and satisfaction. I enjoyed teaching medical students and at the same time I was busy setting up a research laboratory to train graduate students. My first graduate student was a professor from a community college in Los Angeles who wanted to work on a PhD degree. She had taught microbiology and immunology in the community college for many years. She had a lot of research experience. In fact she authored a microbiology textbook used in junior colleges, and had already published dozens of papers in immunology and microbiology. It was quite easy for me to guide her in her research project. Together we chose an immunology project. She completed her course work and research in three years and we were happy to see her receive the PhD degree with a scholarly publication in an immunology journal.[1]

Shortly after I graduated my first PhD student, I was approached by James M. Slater, MD, chair of radiation oncology (now radiation medicine), asking me to consider holding a secondary appointment in his department. Incidentally, Dr. Slater is a world-renowned radiation oncologist (a physician specialized in treating cancer with radiation) and was instrumental in establishing the first and only hospital-based proton treatment center in the world in the 1990s. Dr. Slater wanted me to start an immunology research laboratory to guide physicians and staff in his department to have first-hand research experience. His offer included a premium lab space in Loma Linda University Medical Center (the main university hospital), equipment and supplies for the lab, and a full-time technician. It didn't take me long to consider this offer. In fact I was quite thrilled to accept his offer, knowing that this would provide me with an excellent opportunity to interact with clinicians and staff in the medical center. Since my lab in the microbiology department is only three minutes' walk to the medical center, I felt it would not be difficult for me to oversee both labs. As soon as the immunology lab in the department of radiation medicine was set up we were ready to start our first project. Senior resident Ernest Ngo, MD, and Dr. Slater chose to study the effect of therapeutic irradiation on the immune responses. We enrolled 60 patients into our study. We determined their immune status before, during, and after their treatments. We found that irradiation depressed patients' cellular immunity varying from 48 percent to 64 percent of pretreatment baseline. This depression persisted until about two months after completion of treatment. We also found irradiation of pelvic and abdominal sites showed consistently greater depression than the chest or head and neck group. The degree of depression correlated with clinical outcome. Knowing the immune response of the patients, clinicians may thus be able to adjust the schedule and/or dosages of irradiation to achieve the best results.[2]

I had the opportunity to reconnect with my long-time friend Douglas S. Wong, MD, a professor and radiation oncologist in the department. It has been known that low dose total body irradiation prolonged survival time and improved quality of life of patients with chronic lymphocytic leukemia. We were able to use an animal model called Friend virus-induced leukemia to show that low dose total body irradiation indeed expedited the elimination of cancer cells from animals. When we added an immune modulator, a bacterial vaccine, an even greater elimination of cancer cells was noted.[3] In other words, low dose of radiation and immune modulator showed best results with this RNA virus-induced leukemia. Of course, the results of this study encourage clinicians to use low dose of radiation to treat patients with chronic lymphocytic leukemia and thus greatly minimizing the adverse side effects associated with the treatment.

Graduate students in the microbiology department where I had my primary appointment collaborated with physicians and staff in the radiation medicine department in the hospital in several cancer research projects. One of the major causes of morbidity and mortality in cancer patients is opportunistic fungal infections. This is especially true with leukemias and lymphomas. Of the fungal agents, the most commonly found in association with cancer are *Aspergillus* (a mold fungus), and *Candida* (a yeast-like fungus). However, it is uncertain whether the increase in the incidence of infection is due to lowered resistance caused by cancer or to the anticancer therapy which the patients receive. In animal models, leukemia viruses have been shown to suppress lymphocyte-mediated immune response in mice leading to tumor development and increased risk of opportunistic infections.[4,5] In our lab, we had used a Friend virus-induced leukemia as already mentioned. We now decided to use a chemical carcinogen-induced animal model called L1210 leukemia for the study. The L1210 lymphocytic leukemia was originally obtained in DBA (a special strain) mice after skin painting with a chemical called methycholanthrene.[6] The study was carried out to determine whether animals bearing L1210 leukemia were more susceptible to candida infection in the absence of immunosuppression and to determine also if the L1210 cells suppress the inflammatory response of the animal host. Systemic infection was studied by intravenous injection of *Candida albicans* and checking for the number of candida organisms cultured from the blood and the kidneys. Localized infection was studied by intramuscular injection of *C. albicans* into the thighs and measuring the changes in the thigh size. Compared with tumor-free controls, the intravenous injection resulted in higher counts of *C. albicans* from the blood and the kidneys of tumor-bearing animals. No significant difference in the localized swelling was noted between tumor- and non-tumor-bearing mice with respect to intramuscular injection of *C. albicans*. The results therefore indicate that L1210 leukemia increases susceptibility of tumor-bearing animals to systemic candida infection. The study also showed that L1210 cells reduced the accumulation of neutrophils (white blood cells) and to suppress the normal inflammatory reaction against the fungus. This work was published in *Infection and Immunity*.[7] At about this same time, we also published another paper showing L1210 leukemia differs from virus-induced leukemia in that there is absence of suppression of humoral and cellular immunity, rather there is a suppression of inflammatory reaction in the animals.[8] In subsequent chapter, you will learn that normal inflammatory reaction is a part of the non-specific immunity whereas lymphocyte-mediated humoral and cellular response is a part of the specific immunity. What's the significance? You will find this out when you read the chapter on Cancer Immunology Made Simple.

I consider it a privilege to work closely with Dr. James M. Slater and his associates in the department of radiation medicine for three years when I decided to turn over the responsibility to Daila Gridley, PhD, a new graduate from the department of microbiology. I continued to collaborate with Dr. Gridley and published papers in cancer immunology.[9-11]

Focusing in the lab in microbiology department, I accepted several students who joined me to study the antimicrobial and the anticancer effects of garlic. You might wonder why we chose to study garlic. You see, one of my PhD students, Moses Adetumbi, was from Nigeria. He wanted to conduct research on something that he could continue to research when he returned to his home country. We settled on garlic and were pleased with our choice. We published quite a number of papers with our studies.[12-16] For example, we showed garlic is a broad spectrum antibiotic against not only bacteria, fungi, and parasites, but also viruses. As far as anticancer effects, I am going to devote a good portion of pages to describe them later.

But for now, allow me to fast forward to a new page in my sojourn in Loma Linda. One of the very exciting events during those earlier years at Loma Linda University was my enrollment to be a medical student in the medical school where I was already an associate professor of immunology and microbiology. The medical curriculum at that time was 36 months or three years. But it took me four years to complete the medical degree because I was still teaching during a good portion of the time when I was also a medical student. This dual student/professor role proved interesting and even humorous as I continued to teach microbiology to three classes of medical students who now became my classmates as well. The first hour each day was pathology followed by microbiology in the second hour. I along with my fellow classmates would sit in the auditorium for the pathology class, and then in the second hour I would pop up to the podium to begin my microbiology lecture! Thinking I was trying to be funny, several of my classmates joked with me. Upon realizing that I made no move to sit down, they then advised me to stop making a fool of myself, and a few even tried to pull me down! It took them several minutes to realize that I was indeed their microbiology professor! My students/classmates were happily surprised and proud to accept me as both peer and professor.

My family rejoiced when I completed my medical course and residency training. While in school, my two children were "mad" that their dad spending little time with them even though their mother devoted full time to care for their needs. My daughter often voiced her displeasure to her mother: "Why does daddy have to go to school when he is so old already?" I do not blame her. You see in those few years because I was in school and teaching at the same time, our family did not have long vacations. But they were so glad that I finally made it.

I resumed my full time position as a medical school professor teaching medical and dental students. I also opened my own medical office (clinic) and spending about 10 hours a week in the office. Most of my patients were referred to me by physicians who had been my students. They sent me their toughest patients, those whom they no longer wanted to treat because of poor outcomes. Faced with a caseload of such patients, I discovered that many of their symptoms were related to side effects of drugs rather than to their diagnosis. Furthermore, unhealthy lifestyle choices, particularly dietary, only served to exacerbate their problems. As my wife, a registered dietitian and nutritionist, worked with me, we were soon gratified by our patients' recovery through simple lifestyle changes. Before long, our practice was thriving with patients coming to us from around the U.S., as well as from Europe and Asia.

With the grant from Chan Shun Foundation (an international philanthropic organization established by a successful Chinese business man Dr. Chan Shun), I was able to further expand our cancer research team. Postdoctoral fellows from China, Japan, and the U.S. joined my laboratory. They provided a lot of help for me to train my graduate (MS and PhD) students. We first studied cancer biology and immunology.[17-19] We reported that cancer cells secrete substances that repel our body's cancer-fighting cells, particularly those we call phagocytes (this phenomenon is what I called blindfolding in Chapter 1). As a result, for several years our research was centered on ways to enhance phagocyte activity through various immune stimulants referred to as biological response modifiers or BRMs. We've experimented with live bacterial vaccine, killed bacterial vaccine, and phytochemicals (plant chemicals). Nearly all the BRMs we tested strengthen the body's control against cancer as long as three important conditions are met:

1. The tumor burden has to be low in order for the biological response modifiers to work. In other words, the tumor has to be small—either because it has just begun to grow or because most of it has been removed or destroyed by other means.
2. Dosage and the schedule of administration of biological response modifiers are very important—the lower dosages generally work better than higher dosages. The concept "more is better" does not hold true to the use of these biological response modifiers.
3. The route of administration needs to provide optimal contact between the tumor cells and the biological response modifiers. Local routes near or at the tumor site usually work better than systemic routes.

We also focused our research efforts on the role of nutrition (particularly the use of garlic) in cancer development and prevention. An epidemiological study[20] reported by the People's Republic of China intrigued us. Researchers compared two large populations in Shandong

Province. Residents of the province's Cangshan County enjoyed the lowest death rate due to stomach cancer (3 per 100,000), but the county of Oixia residents had a thirteen fold higher death rate due to the same cancer (40 per 100,000).

What is the difference?

The residents of Cangshan regularly eat 20 grams of garlic per day. The residents of Oixia rarely eat garlic. The study showed that Cangshan residents had lower concentrations of nitrites in their gastric juice than those in Oixia who rarely eat garlic. Apparently garlic protected against the formation of nitrites—the precursors of carcinogens—thus providing a protection against the development of stomach cancer.

Another group of Chinese researchers studied the effect of garlic and diallyl trisulfide (a component of garlic) on the growth of two human stomach cancers in the tissue cultures. They found that garlic and its component inhibited the growth of cancer cells as effectively as did some chemotherapeutic drugs.[21]

What's the implication of these two studies? The first study shows that garlic may well prevent carcinogen-induced cancer; the second shows that it may stop the growth of cancer cells. In other words, it may show promise for both prevention and treatment.

Many other studies bear out the same evidence. Studies conducted by Dr. Michael Wargovich in the Gastrointestinal Oncology Section at the University of Texas's M. D. Anderson Cancer Center showed that organic sulfides, including diallyl sulfide (an important component of garlic), inhibit the development of carcinogen dimethyl hydrazine-induced colon cancer.[22,23] Dr. Wargovich is now with the Hollings Cancer Center, Medical University of South Carolina, continuing his in-depth study of cancer chemoprevention.

Studies by Dr. Sidney Belman at the New York University Medical Center involving mice showed that topical application of garlic oil prevented skin cancer induced by chemical carcinogen dimethyl benzanthracene.[24] Researchers at the University of Minnesota studied mice with benzopyrene-induced stomach cancer. The administration of allyl methyl trisulfide, a constituent of garlic oil, reduced 70 percent of the tumors during the period of the experiment.[25] According to the Minnesota researchers, the component in garlic stimulates an enzyme that protects the stomach from the effects of the carcinogen.

Recently an excellent new book entitled "Anticancer—A New Way of Life" was published by David Servan-Schreiber, MD, PhD. Among many important research studies described in this book is that of Dr. Richard Beliveau, who evaluated some 30 foods regarding their inhibitory activity against cancer cell growth of five human cancers (colon, brain, lung, prostate, and breast). Evidencing the strongest anticancer ability against all these five cancer cell lines was none other than the lowly garlic. Other vegetables showing strong inhibitory activity include leeks, scallions, Brussels sprouts, cabbage, beets, spinach, kale, asparagus, cauliflower, onions, and broccoli.[26] Incidentally, our lab has studied several edible green plants and found them to have strong anticancer activity.[27,28] As a sideline, we also published a paper, based on our clinical observation, showing that green plants can improve the sexual dysfunction in both men and women.[29] The conclusion I can draw here is: Nearly all the edible plants studied so far have anticancer property in varying degrees. These remarkable findings underscore the power of a plant-based diet in fighting cancer. I'll say more about Dr. Servan-Schreiber's book later on. Just a brief introduction about this doctor right now: Dr. Servan-Schreiber had brain cancer, was treated with chemotherapy, after short remission, he had recurrence. He was treated with chemotherapy again and at the same time also changed his diet and lifestyle and he has been well since.

Let me continue some more on my own research. For several years I collaborated with urologists in our medical center in studying bladder cancer in mice. In fact, for two decades I held a secondary appointment in the urology department. Since urology is a part of the big surgery discipline, I actually held a professor of surgery title even though I did not perform any surgery in patients (I did perform surgery in animals).

For our studies of bladder cancer, we used a well-established mouse transitional cell carcinoma model designated as MBT-2, kindly provided by Mark S. Soloway, MD, of the University of Tennessee, Memphis, Tennessee. This tumor was originally derived by feeding C3H/He mice a chemical carcinogen (FANFT), and it has been maintained in the laboratory by serial subcutaneous transplantation in the hind limbs of C3H/He mice. We conducted two studies with one study using tumors transplanted subcutaneously while in the second study tumor cells were introduced into the bladder. Our research looked into the immunotherapy with several known immune enhancing agents including live bacterial vaccine (bacillus Calmette-Guerin or BCG) and killed bacterial vaccine (*Corynebacterium parvum*) and also included garlic extract in our testing. Two landmark papers published in the prestigious *Journal of Urology*[30,31] show that treatment with garlic extract produced the lowest incidence of bladder cancer. The same treatment also resulted in smaller tumors compared with other agents. Garlic apparently stimulates the animal's immune system, particularly, enhancing the activity of macrophages, natural killer cells and lymphocytes, which destroy cancer cells. Our best results occurred when garlic was applied directly to the tumor site. When live vaccine BCG was given systemically, the tumor was not reduced, but it was reduced when the live vaccine was injected locally to the tumor site. The tumor sizes were reduced when either garlic or the killed bacterial vaccine was injected systemically—even greater reduction occurred when the injection was local.

The most remarkable thing about this series of experiments occurred when we examined the tumors under the microscope: what we had originally thought to be smaller tumors treated by garlic or killed bacterial vaccine turned out to be just scar tissues. There were no tumor cells, only debris of dead cells. In other words, the treatments with these two agents actually cured the cancer! The cure was obtained with local injection, not with systemic injection.

Urologist James L. Woolley, MD, was my medical school classmate. He had previously involved in research in my lab. Now with two other urologists, Herbert C. Ruckle, MD, and Robert R. Torrey, MD, proposed a project to study the combined effects of surgery, chemotherapy, and immunotherapy. Again we used mouse transitional cell carcinoma, the same mouse bladder cancer described before, as a model. Mice were transplanted with 500,000 viable tumor cells. Ten to 14 days later when the tumor nodule reached a diameter of five to seven millimeters, it was surgically removed. The mice were then randomized into four groups to receive treatments on days 1, 3, and 5 after surgery: Group 1 treated with saline as control; Group 2 bacterial vaccine *Corynebacterium parvum* (CP); Group 3 chemotherapy with cis-diamminedichloroplatinum (CDDP); and Group 4 combined CP and CDDP. Recurrence of tumor occurred in 70 percent of mice receiving surgery only, in 52 percent of mice receiving CP, in 55 percent receiving CDDP, and in 28 percent receiving combined CP and CDDP. Only the combined immuno- and chemotherapy group showed statistically significant better results compared with the control—surgery only group. The urologists were quite exited with the results that they actually repeated the experiments three times with essentially the same results. In the second part of the experiment, the activities of phagocytes and natural killer cells were determined using animal cells harvested from the peritoneum, spleen, and inguinal lymph nodes. CP or CDDP alone enhanced the phagocyte and natural Killer cell activity. The most significant enhancement was obtained with cells of mice receiving combined CP and CDDP, showing immunotherapy can improve the outcome of chemotherapy. This study was also published in the prestigious *Journal of Urology*.[32]

When we reported results of our animal studies to the general public in European countries, we encountered some objections. Citizens of some European countries did not favor using animals for research. In the U.S. we also encountered resistance on the use of animals. So our group established several *in vitro* (in the test tube) models using tissue culture cells (normal and malignant cancer cells) to continue our studies.[33,34] The two individuals who played the major roles in developing these *in vitro* models were Jeffrey Tosk, a PhD student at that time, and Lin Li, MD, PhD, a postdoctoral fellow from Beijing. This turned out to be a very practical and cost-effective strategy. All the researchers in our lab, both graduate students and postdoctoral fellows, welcomed the *in vitro* models without the use of whole animals.

Using *in vitro* models, PhD student Padma Tadi studied the anticarcinogenic effect of garlic using a chemical carcinogen aflatoxin. Aflatoxin, produced by *Aspergillus* mold, contaminates peanuts, rice, cereal grains, corn, beans, and sweet potatoes, is linked with liver cancer and possibly with other types of cancer. Liver cancer is one of the most prevalent cancers on the worldwide scale, inflicting large populations in Asia and Africa. Aflatoxin is actually a procarcinogen meaning it is not a carcinogen in its natural form. It becomes carcinogenic only when it is metabolized or oxidized into the "epoxide" form in our body. In its epoxide form, it can bind to the nucleic acids (DNA or RNA) or protein molecules in the tissue cells and lead to mutation and cancer formation. We now know that there are several ways our body can prevent the progression of this process. First of all, our body has ways to inhibit the oxidation of aflatoxin to its epoxide. Secondly, if epoxide is formed, our body can inhibit the epoxide from binding to the DNA. Finally, our body has ways to detoxify the epoxide or carcinogenic chemicals by converting them to water-soluble compounds so that they can be excreted. Glutathione conjugates and glucuronide are examples of water-soluble metabolites that can be excreted from our body. Padma Tadi showed that several organosulfur compounds of garlic effectively inhibit the metabolism of aflatoxin to its epoxide. Garlic can inhibit aflatoxin from binding to DNA. Garlic also increases the level of water-soluble metabolites so that the carcinogenic compounds may be detoxified. In other words, Padma's studies demonstrated that garlic can stop cancer by involving it in all three steps of cancer formation. Much of Padma's research was carried out in collaboration with Robert Teel, PhD, professor of physiology and pharmacology. Padma published several papers in peer-reviewed journals[35-37] and received her PhD degree. She went on to conduct research in several universities and recently returned to her alma mater Loma Linda University as a professor in the School of Public Health. Her most recent study deals with lycopene, a red pigmented carotenoid in many fruits and vegetables such as tomatoes. Using a sophisticated technique called proteomic analysis, she reports that lycopene selectively inhibits the growth of human breast cancer cells while exhibits no inhibition for non-cancerous human breast cells.[38]

Before I go on any further, I want to take a moment to talk about two fundamental topics. The first topic deals with the three stages of cancer. The second topic is: What causes cancer? Let me take the first topic: The three stages of cancer are initiation, promotion, and progression. In initiation, an agent enters a normal cell, gets into its nucleus and changes its DNA, and turns this cell into a cancer-prone cell. In other words, now this cell no longer follows the normal growth pattern. When this cell divides, the daughter cells also have the new property, namely, they are also cancer-prone cells. Sooner or later, they grow into a colony or a small tumor in the local site. In promotion, the cancer-prone cells or colony receive special nutrient (promoter food), they then grow into larger colony or tumor and may extend to the adjacent area. Finally, they continue to grow wild and spread to distant area leading to progression. I like Dr. Campbell's analogy on page 48 of his book *The China Study*:[39] the cancer process is similar to planting a lawn. Initiation is when you put the seeds in the soil, promotion is when the grass starts to grow and progression is when the grass gets completely out of control, invading the driveway, the shrubbery and the sidewalk.

What causes cancer? There's no simple answer: many different factors lead to the development of cancer, with chemical carcinogens, radiation, and viruses among those known to us.

More than two hundred years ago, English surgeon Sir Percival Pott noted a high incidence of scrotal cancer among London's chimney sweepers.[40] He correctly pinned fault on exposure to chimney soot—which we now know contains polycyclic hydrocarbons, known to cause cancer in animals. The chemicals in London's chimney soot are the same class of chemicals that filter into the lungs in cigarette smoke, increasing the risk of lung cancer. Scientists suspect that carcinogens result when some of these chemicals combine with foods and bacteria in the large intestine. We'll discuss in great length the potential carcinogens in later chapters.

Another well-known cause of cancer is radiation,[41] and much of what we know about radiation's effects comes from studies of people exposed to ionizing radiation. The list includes physicians and dentists who use X-rays for diagnosis or treatment; uranium miners; and nuclear industry personnel as well as survivors of the nuclear bombings of Hiroshima and Nagasaki. Based on research, we believe that relatively high doses and long period of exposure are necessary to produce cancer.

Still another cause of cancer—both in animals and humans—are viruses. There are numerous examples of animal cancer associated with viruses. Several human cancers are now known to be associated with viruses: Hepatitis B and C viruses associated with liver cancer; Human Papilloma viruses associated with cancer of cervix of uterus; Epstein-Barr virus associated with nasopharyngeal carcinoma and Burkitt's lymphoma; and leukemia associated with human T cell leukemia virus, etc. I believe as time goes on we will discover many more human cancers are associated with viruses.

When Dr. Takeshi Yamasaki, DVM (Doctor of Veterinary Medicine), from Japan's Tokyo University, came to our lab as a postdoctoral research fellow, he brought with him a unique garlic compound called allixin. This is a phytoalexin ("phyto" means plant and "alexin" means to ward off) which is a major weapon used by a plant to fight diseases. Plants do not have a complex immune defense system like animals, nevertheless they utilize chemical defense to protect themselves. Phytoalexins have been described as "stress compounds," because their synthesis is induced by exposure of a plant to certain kinds of stress, such as contact with bacteria, fungi, viruses, insects, and heavy metal chemicals.[42] Understandably, Dr. Yamasaki wanted to find out if this stress compound plays any role in cancer prevention. He employed all the techniques used by Padma Tadi. Lo and behold, he found that this stress compound allixin prevents mutation (change of DNA), inhibits aflatoxin metabolism and its binding to DNA, and enhances water-soluble byproducts to be excreted, just like everything I reported in the last paragraph with other garlic compounds. We submitted his manuscript to a cancer journal,[43] the editor was so excited about this work, that he accepted this paper for publication in five days! Normally, it takes several months to get a paper accepted because it usually involves several referees and a lot of time to complete the critique process.

Another PhD student, Brian Wong, studied four Chinese medicinal herbs.[44-49] *Oldenlandia diffusa* (OD) and *Scutellaria barbata* (SB) are

23

anticancer herbs while *Astragalus membranaceus* (AM) and *Ligustrum lucidum* (LL) are immune enhancers. Brian found all these four herbs significantly inhibited aflatoxin B_1 (AFB_1) binding to DNA, reduced AFB_1-adduct formation, and also decreased the formation of organosoluble metabolites of AFB_1, all these processes stopped the normal liver cells from turning into malignant cancer cells. Brian Wong was (and still is) a very focused and hardworking researcher. During the time in my lab, he authored six scholarly papers and received his PhD degree. Brian went on to become a professor and administrator but continued to study the two Chinese anticancer herbs. In recent years, Brian's daughter Hannah Wong, MD, a pathologist has collaborated with him conducting clinical studies with *Scutellaria barbata* (SB) on cancer patients with promising results.[50]

As a part of the residency training, two urology residents Jerry R. Rittenhouse, MD, and Paul D. Lui, MD, chose to study *Astragalus membranaceus* (AM) and *Ligustrum lucidum* (LL) in reversing macrophage suppression induced by urological cancers. Macrophage is a type of immune cell that can destroy cancer cells. However, macrophage may not be able to carry out its destruction because cancer cells are known to produce soluble factors that can suppress macrophage function. This is what I referred to as the blindfolding tactic used by the cancer cells. Anyway, using the *in vitro* model with cell cultures, we studied two urological cancers—murine renal cell carcinoma (kidney cancer) and murine transitional cell carcinoma (bladder cancer). We first showed that these two cell lines secreted soluble factors that prevented macrophages from killing them. In other words, these cancers can produce factors that blindfold the macrophages and are thus protect themselves from attacks by macrophages. We then demonstrated that in the presence of AM or LL extract, macrophages became active again—being able to attack the cancer cells. These phytochemicals act like removing handkerchiefs that blindfold them. AM and LL have previously been shown to modulate immune response. The data from this study showed that they may also exert their antitumor activity through abolition of cancer-associated macrophage suppression. The study was also published in *Journal of Urology*.[51] This phenomenon was also demonstrated in an animal model (kidney cancer in Balb/c mice) and published in *Cancer Biotherapy*.[52]

Incidentally, *Astragalus membranaceus* (AM) and *Ligustrum lucidum* (LL) are the two most potent immune enhancers. I was introduced to these two herbs by doctors in the largest cancer hospital (Beijing Cancer Hospital) when I visited there 30 years ago. The hospital had a busy outpatient clinic seeing thousands of patients each day. The hospital treated their cancer patients with combined Chinese and western medicines. They had an herbal formula that boosts the immune function, minimizes side effects associated with radiotherapy and chemotherapy. AM and LL are two of the main ingredients in this herbal formula. I brought these two herbs back from China and tested their effects on phagocytes, lymphocytes, and natural killer cells in our *in vitro* models with cell cultures. We were excited to find these two herbs to have very strong synergistic effect meaning the effect of two together is greater than the sum of each by itself. For example, 50 micrograms of AM increased the macrophage activity 4.6 folds, and 50 micrograms of LL increased the macrophage activity 1.5 folds. But when these two were used together they increased the macrophage activity 15.4 folds; while the mathematical sum of AM + LL = 4.6 + 1.5 = 6.1 when used singly.[53] When I reported this finding to the annual convention of the American Society for Microbiology held in New Orleans, reporter John Pope from The Times-Picayune interviewed me and wrote a sensational article titled "Herb duo may work wonders in AIDS battle." Pope's news was picked up by major newspapers in the country, and I was suddenly thrust into the media limelight. A reporter from Washington Post called my office seeking an interview, and I turned him down. But when my son heard about it, he chided me: "Dad, you are indeed an absent-minded professor—you apparently do not know the significance of Washington Post!"

Another news frenzy occurred in the late 1980s when Stephen Rosenberg, MD, PhD, of the National Cancer Institute reported his success with a new type of immunotherapy using recombinant interleukin-2 (rIL-2) and lymphokine activated killer (LAK) cells for treating several advanced terminal cancers such as renal cell carcinoma (kidney cancer) and malignant melanoma (skin cancer). National media reported the exciting news as if the cure for cancer was finally found. However, the success of this treatment was hampered by severe toxicity associated with high doses of rIL-2. The side effects include fluid retention, heart attack, kidney failure, and other life-threatening complications. Urologists Yu Wang, MD, and Roger Hadley, MD, collaborated with postdoctoral fellow Xiao-jiang Qian, MD, in my lab studied the effect of AM extract on the cytotoxicity of rIL-2-generated LAK cells against a murine renal cell carcinoma. Our results indicated a ten-fold potentiation of rIL-2-generated LAK cell cytotoxicity. With AM extract it was possible to reduce the dosage of rIL-2 thus minimized its toxic side effects.[54] This study demonstrated another benefit of AM herbal extract. However, this approach was not put into use as Dr. Rosenberg had at this time terminated his clinical project because all his patients had died after a brief period of remission.

Before I leave this subject, I want to mention some very important lessons we have learned from studying Chinese medicinal herbs. When we found crude herbal extracts with anti-cancer activity, we tried to isolate the active components. Several postdoctoral fellows in my lab had strong chemistry background and were experienced in isolation and purification techniques. They were able to separate a single herb into several purified compounds. They were interested in purified compounds so that they could patent the compounds. What surprised them was when an extract was purified and fractionated, the purified fraction or component often showed no activity or greatly decreased activity compared with the crude extract. In other cases, the isolated component did show strong activity. However, very often this same component also showed increased toxicity. Either way the purified fractions or components were no better than the crude extract. Apparently the different components in the herbal plant have to be together to exert the optimum activity.

In my visits to China in the past ten years, I met several very prominent traditional Chinese medical doctors and herbalists who told me that they had used the two herbs, OD and SB that Brian Wong originally studied, together with diet and lifestyle changes, to cure colon cancer, liver cancer, and stomach cancer. These two herbs are used in the form of concoction, meaning to be prepared by combining diverse ingredients; in this case OD and SB. In China, they use one ounce of SB herb and two ounces of OD herb, extracting them in 20 cups of boiling water by simmering in low heat for three hours. Drink it as herbal tea, one cup two times a day, morning and evening. This quantity of herbal decoction is prepared once a month. In other words, patient takes this decoction only about seven days in a month. I am told that this herbal formula is very potent, so patients take it for one week and rest for three weeks in a month. The Chinese herbalists told me that pharmaceutical companies had tried to purify and isolate the active compounds but found only crude extract works the best. That's why they continue to use decoction of the crude extracts. Several anticancer drugs currently in use were derived from plants or herbs. But because they are so purified, they are indeed very toxic to the body. The anticancer herbs used in China are used in the form of crude extracts. They cannot be patented; but they are non-toxic, inexpensive and affordable to everyone.

A few years ago, my lab was testing a crude extract prepared from the bark of Pacific yew tree (*Taxus brevifolia*) and found the extract to have strong activity against several types of cancers in animals as well as in cultured cancer cells. We were approached by a pharmaceutical company to test the drug Taxol (Paclitaxel), a pure semisynthetic compound isolated originally from Pacific yew tree. We found Taxol effectively stopped the growth of several types of cancers in animals. However, there were many toxic side effects including damaged organs and death which we did not observe with the crude extract. The company advised us not to publish the data and we complied. Meanwhile Taxol continued to be a popular anticancer drug for breast cancer, lung cancer, ovarian cancer, and prostate cancer. It prolongs the patients' lifespan from several months to a few years. However, it is a very expensive drug costing thousands of dollars each dose. It also has a lot of side effects. I just wonder if crude extract of the bark of Pacific yew will also stop the cancer in humans as we have demonstrated it in animals. It will certainly cost much less and possibly with little or no toxic side effects. Of course, this is not something that will interest the pharmaceutical companies. That's why no clinical studies have been conducted with crude plant extracts. I just checked the current Physicians' Desk Reference (PDR). Taxol or Paclitaxel is not listed there. Instead, a good section is devoted to Taxotere—the newest anticancer drug related to Taxol. It is recommended for breast cancer, head and neck cancer, lung cancer, prostate cancer and stomach cancer. There are several pages of warnings on the use of Taxotere including sudden death. If patients read these warnings, it is most likely they will consider the matter twice before consenting to use it.

When Chinese medicinal herbs are used in the form of a concoction it is called an herbal formula. An herbal formula must be effective for its intended use and must also be free of toxic side effect. Chinese herbal formula usually consists of two or more herbs. According to the Chinese herbal principle, every herbal formula must have four components. These four components or ingredients are known as Imperial (君), Ministerial (臣), Assistant (佐), and Servant (使). The major ingredient, the Imperial, is the Emperor Herb that is primarily responsible for dealing with the disorder under treatment. The subsidiary ingredient— the Minister—assists the Emperor herb by promoting its action. The Assistant lessens the imperial herb's side effects or limits its actions, particularly if the imperial herb possesses toxic properties. Finally, the Servant ensures the efficient delivery of the imperial herb and also renders the formula more palatable. In order to have these four components an herbal formula is usually made of several herbs, at least two herbs as in OD and SB. Very often an herbal formula may consist of four or more herbs. The goal is to have an herbal formula that is most effective for the clinical entity and at the same time with minimum or no toxic side effects.

CHAPTER 3

MORE BASIC
NUTRITIONAL RESEARCH

Amber R. Buz'Zard, PhD conducted both her master's and doctoral research in my lab at Loma Linda University School of Medicine. She had a special interest in ovarian cancer and expressed her desire to investigate this specific type of cancer. She did a very thorough literature search and convinced our group that this is a worthwhile area of research. Ovarian cancer is the sixth most common occurring cancer in women. Symptoms are often vague and easily confused with other disorders, resulting in advanced stage detection in more than two-thirds of cases. Thus it accounts for more deaths than any other cancers of the female reproductive system.[1] The symptoms include swelling of the abdomen (due to a mass or accumulation of fluid), unusual vaginal bleeding, pelvic pressure, back pain, leg pain, and digestive problems such as gas, bloating, indigestion or lingering stomach pain.[2] When ovarian cancer is found early at a localized stage, about 90 percent of patients live longer than five years after diagnosis and treatment. However, less than 25 percent of cases are found at this stage, with the majority being found in the later stages. The five year survival rate, with treatment, for stage III is 20 to 40 percent and roughly 11 percent for stage IV.[1]

An effective chemopreventive agent is urgently needed to combat this deadly disease. The most useful compounds for this purpose will have minimal long-term toxicity, while significantly reducing cancer incidence, delaying cancer onset or preventing cancer progression.

When Dr. Buz'Zard proposed to study ovarian cancer, our lab no longer used animal models. Instead, we were using *in vitro* tissue culture cells for all our studies. Dr. Buz'Zard decided to use human ovarian cancer cell lines and normal non-malignant ovarian cells for her studies. Basically, she used three types of tissue culture cell lines: normal, benign, and malignant ovarian cells of human origin. Her phenomenal networking abilities put in touch with scientists all over the world. She was able to find out where to get these human ovarian cells. She purchased several cell lines from the American Type Culture Collection, Manassas, Virginia. Two very important cell lines not available commercially were donated to her by Dr. Louis Dubeau at the University of Southern California and Dr. Hitoshi Okamura at Kumamoto University, Japan. The potential chemopreventive agent she chose to study was called Pycnogenol® consisting of water-soluble bioflavonoids extracted from the bark of the French maritime pine, donated to us by Horphag Research Laboratory, Geneva, Switzerland. These bioflavonoids are found in many fruits and vegetables in varying concentrations. We chose to use Pycnogenol® because it is a standardized product that will yield consistent results.

What are her findings?

She found Pycnogenol® selectively toxic to malignant ovarian germ cells in a dose-dependent manner by causing these cells to undergo apoptosis. Apoptosis means programmed cell death. In other words, the bioflavonoids cause the cancer cells to commit suicide. Interestingly, Pycnogenol® is not toxic to normal ovarian cells, and only slightly toxic to the benign ovarian tumor cells. Thus this compound meets criteria of an ideal chemopreventive agent mentioned earlier.[3]

In another of her studies, talc was found to induce neoplastic or malignant transformation of human ovarian cells in the tissue cultures. Pycnogenol® reduces talc-induced transformation showing again that this phytochemical can prevent cancer development.[4] It is tempting to suggest that bioflavonoids in foods may do the same in preventing and reversing ovarian cancer in human bodies. Our observational research from various educational centers using nutritional therapy does seem to suggest that this may indeed just be possible.

For example, The Gerson Institute in San Diego, California has been teaching plant-based diet to help people to overcome diseases and to regain health. A few years ago a woman with ovarian cancer asked her oncologist to give her names of 20 patients he had treated. She phoned these patients and found out 18 of them had already died. She also asked The Gerson Institute to give her 20 names of ovarian cancer women who have been treated by nutrition therapy. She phoned and was able to speak to 18 women who are living and still cancer free.[5] In this case it seems nutrition does play a beneficial role in the survival of ovarian cancer.

CHAPTER 4

ADVENTIST
HEALTH STUDY

Loma Linda University, affiliated with the Seventh-day Adventist Church, has a School of Public Health which over the past three decades has been conducting ongoing research comparing the health of the Seventh-day Adventists with that of the general population. These studies, funded by the National Institutes of Health, resulted in meaningful epidemiological findings with far-reaching implications.

A good portion of the materials in this chapter is taken from a paper I published in the fall 2007 issue of *Spectrum*,[1] a journal of Adventist Forum.

The November 2005 issue of *National Geographic* magazine reports that Seventh-day Adventists are among the longest-lived people in the world. Citing studies by Gary Fraser, MB, ChB, PhD and his associates at Loma Linda University, the article shows that Adventists in California lived four to ten years longer than the average Californian. Adventists' habits of consuming whole grains, fruits, vegetables and nuts while avoiding red meats, tobacco and alcohol lower their risk of developing cancer and heart disease. Studies also noted that Adventists increase their chances for long life by associating closely with those practicing a similar lifestyle.

Three important publications from the Adventist Health Study led to the favorable report in *National Geographic*. First is a paper titled "Ten Years of Life–Is It a Matter of Choice?" published in *Archives of Internal Medicine* by Drs. Gary Fraser and David Shavlik from the School of Public Health, Loma Linda University.[2] In this paper, the expected length of life of California Adventists (78.5 years for men, 80.2 years for vegetarian men; 82.3 years for women, 84.8 years for vegetarian women) is compared with the populations in 10 countries including

Australia (73.9 years for men, 80.0 years for women), Canada (73.0 years for men, 79.7 years for women), Japan (75.9 years for men, 81.8 years for women), and U.S. general population (73 years for men, 79.7 years for women). Japanese have often been described as the longest-lived population, but as shown in Table 1, California Adventists outlive the Japanese on average. Another highlight of this paper shows that among California Adventists, vegetarian men and women out-lived their non-vegetarian counterparts.

Table 1

Expected Length of Life in Years: California Adventists Compared with International Populations

Country	Men	Women
Australia	73.9	80.0
Canada	73.0	79.7
Denmark	72.0	77.7
Finland	70.9	78.9
Iceland	75.7	80.3
Japan	75.9	81.8
New Zealand	71.6	77.6
Norway	73.4	79.8
United Kingdom	71.9	77.6
United States	73.0	79.7
California Adventists	78.5	82.3
Calif. Adventists-Vegetarians	80.2	84.8

Source: Gary E. Fraser and David J. Shavlik, "Ten Years of Life: Is It a Matter of Choice?" *Archives of Internal Medicine* 161 (July 2001):1645–52.

The second study is titled "Cancer incidence among California Seventh-day Adventists, 1976-1982" by Dr. Fraser's group, published in the *American Journal of Clinical Nutrition*.[3] This study compared cancer incidence among California Adventists with that of the general population in Connecticut. The comparison was made by calculating the standardized morbidity ratios (SMRs). Table 2 has some interesting findings taken from this study. There were a total of 598 cases of cancer observed in California Adventist males during this period (1976-1982), while the expected incidence rate for the reference population was 814 cases, resulting in an SMR of 0.73 for cancers of all sites for Adventist men (598 divided by 814 = 0.73). This difference is statistically significant.

Table 2

Observed and Expected Cancer Incidence in Adventist Males, 1976–1982

Site or type cancer	Observed (O)	Expected (E)	SMR of (O/E)
All cancers	598	814	0.73*
Esophagus	0	14	0.00*
Stomach	15	30	0.50*
Colon	62	98	0.64*
Rectum	25	49	0.51*
Bronchus and lung	41	162	0.25*
Melanoma of skin	23	13	1.77
Prostate	186	149	1.25*
Bladder	37	62	0.59*
Kidney	8	21	0.37*
Brain	15	10	1.49

Source: P. K. Mills, W. L. Beeson, R. L. Phillips, and G. E. Fraser, "Cancer Incidence among California Seventh-day Adventists, 1976–1982," *American Journal of Clinical Nutrition* 59 (May 1994):1136S–1142S.

* Asterisk denotes statistically significant difference.

A third study published by Dr. Fraser, titled "Association between diet and cancer, ischemic heart disease, and all-cause mortality in non-Hispanic White California Seventh-day Adventists," also appeared in the *American Journal of Clinical Nutrition*.[4] This study compared three groups of California Adventists: vegetarians who ate no meat, fish, or poultry; semi-vegetarians who ate meat, fish, or poultry less than one time per week; and non-vegetarians who ate these foods more than once a week. The average body weight for vegetarian, semi-vegetarian, and non-vegetarian men were 77 kilograms (kg) (169.4 pounds), 80 kg (176 lbs.), and 83 kg (182.6 lbs.), respectively. For women, the numbers were 63 kg (138.6 lbs.), 66 kg (145.2 lbs.), and 69 kg (151.8 lbs.), respectively. In both men and women, vegetarians are thinner than non-vegetarians.

Despite the seemingly good news, a closer look at some of the data raises some troubling questions. For example, CL was a dynamic pastor who led a flourishing 300-member congregation flourished with 50 percent of the membership made up of young families. He cared for his health through regular exercise and a lacto-ovo-vegetarian (which includes dairy products and eggs). One day while jogging, CL succumbed to a massive heart attack. He was only 42 years old and left behind a wife and two small children. How did such a healthy person die at such a young age?

Not long ago, a 46-year-old physician suffered a heart attack and died after two weeks in a coronary intensive care unit. He had been a lacto-ovo-vegetarian all his life, and yet he died too young. Why?

JL, a minister's wife who had been a lacto-ovo-vegetarian all her life, recently died of ovarian cancer after undergoing surgery and chemotherapy. Why didn't her diet spare her from ovarian cancer?

One possible answer to the above questions is that eggs and diary in the diet may be the very culprit. Numerous studies have now shown that dairy products contribute to cancers, heart disease, diabetes, osteoporosis, and a host of other maladies of affluent societies. In the Adventist Health Study, over one-third of California Adventist vegetarians consumed eggs and dairy. Only about 4% of the respondents in the study reported a totally plant based diet

Let us look at some specific cancers. As Table 2 shows, the SMRs for cancers of the esophagus, stomach, colon, rectum, lung, bladder, and kidney in Adventist men are 0.00, 0.50, 0.64, 0.51, 0.25, 0.59, and 0.37, respectively. All these numbers are statistically significant indicating Adventist men indeed have significantly lower incidence of these various cancers as compared to the general male population. However, the SMRs for cancers of the skin, prostate, and brain among Adventist men are 1.77, 1.25, and 1.49, respectively, which means that they actually have higher incidence of skin, prostate, and brain cancer. Particularly disconcerting is the higher incidence of prostate cancer. We could speculate that the culprit again may be the lacto-ovo-vegetarian diet. Numerous studies have now shown that dairy food is the primary contributer to prostate cancer. A 2001 Harvard review[6] of the research could not be more convincing: A positive association between dairy products and prostate cancer was found in 12 out of 14 case-control studies and in seven of nine cohort studies.

More recently, two studies published in the *American Journal of Epidemiology* revealed a positive correlation between low-fat and nonfat milk consumption and the risk of prostate cancer. One study looked at questionnaires completed by 82,483 men in the Multiethnic Cohort Study, 4,404 of whom developed prostate cancer over a mean follow-up period of eight years. Consuming one cup or more per day of low-fat or nonfat milk showed a positive association for developing prostate cancer.[7] The other study assessed food frequency questionnaires from 293,888 participants of the National Institutes of Health-AARP Diet and Health Study; of these, 10,180 men had prostate cancer. Skim milk consumption at two or more servings per day was positively associated with an increased risk of advanced prostate cancer.[8]

Let us look at Table 3 regarding cancer incidence in Adventist females, studied during 1976-1982. For Adventist women there were a total of 862 cases of various types of cancer while the expected number of cases was 937, resulting in an SMR of 0.92. In other words, the incidence of all cancers for SDA women is 92% of that of the reference population, or 8% less; the difference here is not statistically significant. The SMRs of stomach cancer, colon cancer and lung cancer are 0.16, 0.76 and 0.36; all of these are statistically significant. For breast cancer, the SMR is 0.91. This means when 100 women in the general population have breast cancer, there are 91 Adventist women who also suffer breast cancer. The difference here is not significant from the standpoint of statistics.

Table 3

Observed and Expected Cancer Incidents in Adventist Females,
1976–1982

Site or type cancer	Observed (O)	Expected (E)	SMR of (O/E)
All cancers	862	937	0.92
Stomach	4	24	0.16*
Colon	95	126	0.76*
Rectum	37	52	0.71
Bronchus and lung	27	76	0.36*
Melanoma of skin	24	14	1.71*
Breast	231	254	0.91
Cervix of uterus	32	20	1.60*
Uterus	129	68	1.91*
Ovary	47	36	1.29
Genital	208	135	1.54*

Source: P. K. Mills, W. L. Beeson, R. L. Phillips, and G. E. Fraser, "Cancer Incidence among California Seventh-day Adventists, 1976–1982," *American Journal of Clinical Nutrition* 59 (1994):1136S–42S.

*Asterisk denotes statistically significant difference.

The SMRs of Adventist women for cancers of the skin, cervix, uterus, ovary, and genitals are 1.71, 1.60, 1.91, 1.29, and 1.54, respectively. In other words, Adventist women have higher incidence of these cancers than non-Adventist women. Particularly disturbing are cancers of the female reproductive system including life-threatening ovarian cancer. Again, like prostate cancer in men, dairy products may be a particular culprit for ovarian cancer. As a part of the more recent Adventist Health Study looking into dietary risk factors for ovarian cancer, researchers at Loma Linda University reported an increased risk of ovarian cancer for meat and cheese intake.[9] A review of a meta-analysis of epidemiological studies published by researchers at the National Institute of Environmental Medicine, Karolinska Institute, Sweden concludes that high intakes of dairy foods and lactose (milk sugar) increase the risk of ovarian cancer.[10] This report about milk sugar is of interest. Most studies indicate milk protein (casein) rather than milk sugar (lactose), contributes to cancer development. Many people use low-fat or nonfat milk, thinking it is preferable to whole milk. What they do not realize is that the removal of fat actually increases the concentration of milk protein and lactose (milk sugar). In other words, low-fat milk contains more protein and sugar than the whole milk. Greater concentration of milk protein contributes to various forms of cancer such as breast and liver cancer. Greater concentration of milk sugar is now linked to ovarian cancer and prostate cancer. Lactose or milk sugar is broken down in the body to a simple sugar called galactose, which is believed to be damaging to the ovaries, reducing fertility and increasing cancer risk.[11]

Back to the third study by Dr. Fraser's group. Looking at the relationship between beef consumption and fatal heart attack, the study compared three groups of Adventist men: those who never consume beef, those who consume beef three times a week, and those who consume beef more than three times a week. The results showed that those who consumed beef three times a week had nearly twice (1.93 times) fatal heart attacks than those who never consumed beef, and those who consumed beef more than three times a week had 2.31 times greater incidence of fatal heart attack than those who never consumed beef. By contrast, women who consumed beef had a slightly lower incidence of fatal heart attack as compared with those who did not consume beef. Hormones in beef may account for this difference, as it has been well documented that premenopausal women have lower incidence of heart attack because of protection from female hormones.

Another fascinating finding from this study is the higher incidence and relative risk of several common cancers in non-vegetarian Adventists as compared to vegetarian Adventists. For example, the relative risk for colon cancer in non-vegetarians is 1.88 (nearly two times) greater than the vegetarians. This difference is highly significant. The incidence of diabetes and high blood pressure in non-vegetarians is also twice as high as in the vegetarians.

In summary, these published reports from the Adventist Health Study reveal the following:

1. Adventists have longer average life span than the general population.
2. Adventists have lower incidence of several cancers compared to those who are not Adventists.
3. Adventist men have greater incidence of prostate cancer than the general population.
4. Adventist women have greater incidence of reproductive system cancers compared to the general population.
5. Adventist women have just about as much breast cancer as the general population.
6. Beef consumption increases the chances of a fatal heart attack in Adventist men.
7. Adventist vegetarians are almost two times more likely to avoid colon cancer, diabetes and high blood pressure than Adventist non-vegetarians.

So what are the implications of the studies cited in *National Geographic* magazine? For those Adventists who have benefited from the diet and lifestyle, the news is confirmatory. But what about the many who have succumbed to heart attack and cancer? Can something be done to reduce the number of premature deaths among the Adventists? The answer is YES.

The lacto-ovo-vegetarian diet has served its intended purpose well for many decades when cow's milk and dairy products were produced by animals raised in farms free from contaminations of hormones, pesticides, carcinogens, and drugs. Today, milk and dairy products are "manufactured" in cattle factories rather than farms. Numerous studies have linked fats in cow's milk and dairy products to heart attacks and strokes. There are more than 2000 published papers studying the relationship between cow's milk and cancers with a large number of papers showing a link to breast cancer, colon cancer, ovarian cancer, prostate cancer, leukemia and lymphoma. Cow's milk is also linked to multiple sclerosis, Alzheimer's disease, and osteoporosis. Most Adventists consume dairy products and eggs. Since they do not eat meats, they may actually consume more animal products in the form of milk and cheese than meat eaters. This may explain the higher incidence among Adventists of prostate and ovarian cancers, both of which are particularly linked to dairy products.

In my practice, patients with elevated prostate specific antigen (PSA) often consult me for a treatment plan. Their doctors suspect prostate cancer and recommend surgery, radiotherapy or chemotherapy. I usually tell them: regardless of what form of treatment they choose to receive, they need to greatly cut down the intake of animal products including dairy. Very often their PSA drops down to normal range within two to three months after their dietary change.

In 2005, Dean Ornish, MD, and his associates at the University of California, San Francisco, School of Medicine published a remarkable study in the *Journal of Urology*.[12] Enrolled in the study were 93 men diagnosed with early stage of prostate cancer confirmed by biopsy and had chosen not to undergo conventional cancer treatment. The control group consisted of 49 men who made no dietary or lifestyle changes but rather merely relied on regular surveillance of the disease. The 44 men in the experimental group were asked to make comprehensive diet and lifestyle changes (vegetarian diet, regular exercise, and stress management). Twelve months later, six patients in control group had to undergo conventional treatment because of a 6% increase in PSA and progression of the disease. In contrast, those in the experimental group experienced a 4% decrease in PSA. But even more impressive is the comparison of lab tests between the two groups. Those who made dietary and lifestyle changes tested out to have blood that was eight times stronger in stopping the growth of prostate cancer cells. It was found that the more diligently these men had followed Dr. Ornish's lifestyle changes, the more active their blood in arresting cancer cell growth.

Six year ago, my wife and I conducted lifestyle medicine seminars in a health center in China. We met a lady physician suffering from the deadly ovarian cancer. Even after two rounds of chemotherapy, her cancer continued to spread. Her doctors gave her up to die. She was encouraged by her friends to live out her final days at the health center where she could enjoy the simple plant-based diet, exercise program, massage, and hydrotherapy. In our lectures we mentioned the link between cow's milk and ovarian cancer. Shocked upon learning that, she revealed to us that she had been drinking copious amounts of cow's milk in the past 10 years; and while receiving chemotherapy, she had been urged by her doctors to even greater milk consumption. At the health center, however, soy milk rather than cow's milk was served. During her two months at the center, instead of dying, she steadily improved. Six months later she called to inform the health center staff that her oncologists in Beijing and Shanghai were amazed that no cancer could be detected. Last year when we were in China, we found her to be totally different from eight years ago when we first saw her. She was now vibrant, energetic, and still cancer free.

I mentioned earlier *The China Study* by Dr. Colin Campbell. In his study of liver cancer in animals, he exposed animals to aflatoxin, a liver carcinogen. Then he divided the animals into three groups with the following: 1) a diet containing 5% milk protein (casein), 2) a diet containing 20% milk protein, and 3) a diet containing 20% plant (soy) protein. None of the animals fed 20% soy protein developed liver cancer, nor did the 5% milk protein-fed animals, but all of the animals fed 20% milk protein developed liver cancer. In another experiment, Dr. Campbell reported that he was able to turn on and turn off cancer— when the diet of cancer ridden animals was switched from 20% milk protein to 5% milk protein, the cancer gradually disappeared. But when the cancer-free animals originally on 5% milk protein were switched to 20% milk protein, sooner or later they developed cancer.

Dr. Campbell and his associates then went to the Philippines to study liver cancer in children. Many children had been infected with hepatitis B virus, and many possibly had been exposed to the liver carcinogen aflatoxin as well. Yet only those whose diet was rich in animal protein suffered liver cancer.

Dr. Campbell's study showing that cancer can be turned on and off is especially intriguing to me, as I have personally known individuals with cancers of breast, colon, and prostate who became cancer free when they changed to a plant-based diet. I also know three friends whose colon cancer went into remission after switching to a plant-based diet, only to have the cancer return within six months to one year after they resumed an animal-based diet.

Several knowledgeable organizations in the U.S. and abroad are currently promoting a plant-based diet for prevention of heart attack, stroke, cancer, and a host of chronic degenerative diseases. For example, the Physicians Committee for Responsible Medicine (www.pcrm.org) mentioned earlier, for over two decades has been recommending a plant-based diet. As Dr. Neal Barnard, president of Physicians' Committee for Responsible Medicine, advised: "The link between diet and cancer is too big to be ignored and it is more critical than ever that you and your loved ones have the resources available to learn how your diet can play a key role in the prevention of cancer. And, if cancer is diagnosed, that the foods you eat can increase your chances for survival."[13] Dr. Barnard has written a number of books dealing with the health benefits of a plant-based diet. Recently with dietitian Jennifer Reilly, he coauthored *The Cancer Survivor's Guide—Foods that Help You Fight Back,* a very practical book to have in the library.

CHAPTER 5

CANCER IMMUNOLOGY MADE SIMPLE

Immunology is the study of the immune function also known as immunity or host defense. In this chapter, I would like to present to you the immunity, particularly, as it is related to cancer.

There are two types of immunity: the native and the adaptive immunity. The native immunity is also referred to as the natural immunity or innate immunity. The adaptive immunity is also known as the acquired immunity.

The native immunity is the type that you and I are borne with whereas the adaptive or acquired immunity is the type that you and I acquire in our life time. One of the unique properties of the acquired immunity is that it is *specific* because it is *antigen-driven.* Let me illustrate. If a child has measles, in about two weeks his body will develop immunity against the measles virus which is the *antigen.* But this immunity is specific for measles virus only, not for chickenpox virus or German measles virus. Note here the acquired immunity becomes effective about two weeks after the first contact with the intruder (the measles virus in this instance); it has no effect against the virus when it first encounters the virus. The native immunity, on the other hand, can attack the intruder right away upon first contact. Furthermore, it is *non-specific* because it is not driven by an antigen. Therefore, the native immunity is effective against a variety of different bacteria, fungi and viruses, and different unwanted substances such as different types of cancer cells.[1] When teaching medical students, I would usually ask at this point, "Which of these two types of immunity is more versatile?" Of course, the native or natural or innate immunity is indeed more versatile. That is one of the reasons that my associates and I have devoted more than three decades to study natural immunity.

Another vital difference between these two types of immunity is that acquired immunity has memory. Let me illustrate using the above example of the child with measles. In about two weeks he develops immunity against the virus but the immunity wanes in a few months or a year. But if a few years later, this same child encounters measles virus again, in a matter of 48 hours or less, his body will mount a strong immunity against the measles virus. Remember the first time it took two weeks for the immunity to develop but this time it takes only two days. Why? Because his body has memory cells that recognize the virus, and immediately they elicit a response to activate the immune system! The native immunity does not have memory. It does not need memory because the cells in the native immunity system are always there to protect us. All the time, day and night.

Our skin and mucous membranes are a part of our native immunity. The normal microbial flora (those germs which reside in our body surfaces and cavities) are also a part of the native immunity; they actually protect us from foreign intruders. Unfortunately, the indiscriminate use of antibiotics kills our friendly microbes and destroys a part of our native immunity. Other factors in native immunity include complement, a protein that plays an important role in fighting some of the germs; and interferons—the glycoproteins made by our cells after a virus infection. Interferons interfere with virus growth. Once when the interferons are produced, they are effective against various other viruses in addition to the original virus that had induced its production. Because their action is non-specific, they are also a part of the native immunity. We also have defensins—proteins secreted by neutrophils (white blood cells) that kill bacteria; lactoferrin, an iron binding protein that inhibits bacterial growth; and lysosomal enzymes that break down cell walls of bacteria and thus destroying them.[2]

Then, there are four types of cells that are parts of the native immunity: neutrophils, monocytes, macrophages, and natural killer cells. Natural killer cells are essential in killing cancer cells. Just about every day a few of our normal body cells are transformed into cancer cells. Fortunately, these cancer cells are destroyed by natural killer cells right away before they have a chance to increase in number.

Natural killer cells are special members in the immune system. Like all other white blood cells, they patrol continually in our body in search of viruses and cancer cells. But while other cells like B cells and T cells need previous exposure to disease agents in order to recognize and combat them, natural killer cells do not need prior introduction to an intruder in order to mobilize it. As soon as they detect an enemy, they gather around the intruder, seeking membrane-to-membrane contact. Once they make contact, natural killer cells release their vesicles—the chemical weapons containing perforins and granzymes that damage the intruder's membrane causing it to rupture and die.[3] The deflated remains are then digested by macrophages, which are the garbage collectors of the immune system and are always found in the wake of natural killer cells.[3,4]

The adaptive or acquired immunity is subdivided into humoral immunity consisting of B lymphocytes and cellular immunity consisting of T lymphocytes. B lymphocytes respond to various stimuli by producing antibodies, which help fight off many common infections. We now recognize at least four subtypes of T lymphocytes: the helper T lymphocytes, which are always ready to help other cells; the cytotoxic T lymphocytes, whose main job is to control foreign invaders; the suppressor T lymphocytes, which act as military police to ensure that other cell types do not transgress their limit. The fourth type of T lymphocytes has the ability to destroy parasites. Unfortunately, it is also involved in certain undesirable allergic reactions such as contact dermatitis in persons allergic to poison oak or cosmetics.

There are two types of lymphoid organs—the Primary and the Secondary. The Primary Lymphoid Organs are where lymphocytes are manufactured—like the factories. The Secondary Lymphoid Organs are the sites where the activities of lymphocytes are being carried out—like the market place. The two Primary Lymphoid Organs are the thymus—a small organ behind the breast bone, where the T lymphocytes (T cells) are developed, and the bone marrow, particularly abundant in the long bones where the B lymphocytes (or B cells) are derived. So the T lymphocytes are thymus-derived lymphocytes and B lymphocytes are bone marrow-derived lymphocytes. The Secondary

Lymphoid Organs include the spleen situated in the left side of the belly; and the lymph nodes scattered in strategic places throughout our body.

Now let me describe to you the functions of various immune cells. Neutrophils, monocytes and macrophages are called phagocytes ("phago" meaning "eating" in Greek) because they "eat up" bacteria, viruses, parasites, and any unwanted particles in our body. The unwanted particles may include cancer cells. B cells are needed to fight bacteria, viruses, and parasites, but not on first contact with these agents. B cells need to make antibodies which take time and complex process. T cells are important in fighting viruses, intracellular microbes, and cancer cells. Like B cells, they do not attack intruders on first contact. T cells also need time and complex process to develop their ammunition. Like T cells, natural killer cells are also important for fighting viruses and cancer cells.[5] Unlike T cells, the action of natural killer cells is instant upon contact. As mentioned before, every day a few normal cells in our body may turn into cancer cells. They are usually destroyed by natural killer cells and/or phagocytes right away. Someone has said that every person has cancer cells in the body but not everyone suffers cancer. Thanks to the defense mechanism mediated by our body's natural immunity.

If our immune system is in prime condition we can fight cancer easily. However, when our immune system is weakened, a few cancer cells can eventually develop into deadly cancer.

Today we know that lifestyle habits are major causes of cancer, coronary heart disease, infections, and as well as a host of other diseases. How we live has a direct influence, either positively or negatively, on our immune system. What are some of the lifestyle habits that may weaken the immune system? I have used the two words "FAT CAT" to describe the six most important factors that may suppress the immune function. What is the "**FAT CAT?**"

F refers to food (rich food with fats and refined sugars), **A** for anxiety (stress), and **T** for toxicity (chemicals and drugs). **CAT** refers to three legalized drugs used by the general public: Caffeine, Alcohol, and Tobacco.[6,7]

Let's begin with **F** or food. Both the American Cancer Society and the National Cancer Institute have recommended a reduction of total fat intake and an increase of vegetables, fresh fruits, and whole grains.[8,9] For example, the risk of breast cancer doubles in women who have high levels of trans fat in their blood.[10] Interestingly, our immune cells cannot tolerate high fat either. High fat makes these cells lazy so that they cannot function at full capacity. On the other hand, green and yellow leafy vegetables and fresh fruits contain special vitamins, and minerals that make healthy immune cells. With a good diet, our immune cells are alert, active, and responsible in carrying out both their defensive and offensive functions. When the immune cells are healthy, enemies such as pathogenic bacteria, viruses, and cancers have less chance to survive.

Refined sugars really hurt the immune function. A few years ago my colleagues and I published a study showing that refined sugar impairs the function of neutrophils, the type of white blood cells that destroy disease-producing bacteria.[11] We now know that refined sugar lowers our resistance and make us vulnerable to all types of common infections. Children catch colds after eating rich desserts or candy. When mothers eliminate sweets from their children's diet, these youngsters no longer suffer frequent colds. I teach my students that 80 to 90 percent of the time when children get upper-respiratory infections (sore throat, sinus, or ear infection), it is because of a virus. A culture should be taken. If the culture does not show pathogenic bacteria, the child should not be given antibiotics. Antibiotics do not kill viruses, but will kill the good bacteria and will further lower the person's resistance. The best treatment and prevention for colds is a good diet with no junk food and sweets. Today we also recognize that refined sugar feeds cancer. Cancer cells consume eighteen times more sugar than normal cells because they have more glucose receptors on the cell surface. Elevated blood sugar (glucose) is associated with leukemia, and cancers of esophagus, larynx, stomach, colon, rectum, liver, bile duct, pancreas, prostate, bladder and brain. The higher the blood sugar level, the higher is the incidence of these cancers.[12]

A for anxiety (stress) – Studies in the 1960s suggested that stress may affect the immune system. Early studies carried out in animals showed that either physical or psychological stress increases blood levels of corticosteroid, or "stress hormone." The stress hormone in turn causes the depression of all immune cells—B cells, T cells, natural killer (NK) cells, and phagocytes. Human studies done in the past few years support this hypothesis.[13] For example, medical students have decreased NK cell activity and decreased helper T lymphocytes just before a major examination.[14] Sleep deprivation, as a stress, has been shown to decrease T lymphocyte function.[15] Stress per se, however, is not necessarily detrimental to the person or the immune system. Rather, what matters is how the individual copes with the stress. Studies have shown that breast cancer patients who cope poorly with stress often have a poor prognosis, and vice versa.[16]

T for toxicity—particularly toxic chemicals and drugs—recreational drugs, over-the-counter drugs and prescription drugs all may negatively affect the immune system. Marijuana, for example, suppresses the immune system, impairs reproduction, produces respiratory disease, and increases the risk of lung cancer. Marijuana has been shown to depress T lymphocyte and macrophage activity.[17] Cocaine suppresses cytotoxic T lymphocytes, natural killer cells, and phagocytes,[18] all of which are essential in fighting cancer. In addition to these so-called recreational drugs, bear in mind that over-the-counter as well as prescription drugs also harm the immune system. I always encourage my patients to read the inserts that come with the drugs paying special attention to the intended use and possible adverse side effects. Many drugs may show adverse reactions such as leukopenia (decrease of white blood cells), granulocytopenia (decrease of disease-fighting cells called granulocytes) or marrow hypoplasia (decrease of bone marrow where immune cells are manufactured).

C for coffee–caffeine has been shown to lower the response of T lymphocytes in both men and women. Both B cell and natural killer cell activity is decreased during coffee consumption.[19] These cells are needed for antibody production and natural defense, respectively. What many people may not be aware of is that caffeine is also present in many soft drinks, chocolate, and over-the-counter drugs.

A for alcohol – Most of us are aware of the horrendous problems associated with alcoholism. A computer search of relevant literature reveals more than 100 scientific reports published in recent decades showing that alcohol consumption down-regulates the immune system.[20] Several studies show that alcohol profoundly decreases the normal function of B lymphocytes, cytotoxic T lymphocytes, natural killer cells, and phagocytes.[21,22] If you can imagine how a person behaves under the influence of alcohol—careless, indifferent, unsteady—that is how researchers discovered immune cells behave when they are bathed in an environment of alcohol. They don't seem to care about their responsibilities.

How much alcohol is needed to produce a harmful effect? Antibody production levels dropped more than threefold in individuals consuming only two drinks. In other words, after just two drinks, your antibody defenses operate at less than one third of the normal. In another study, cytotoxic T lymphocytes lost their resistance to viruses after individuals drank an average of four beers. The immune down-regulating effect of alcohol persisted for days, even after the alcohol was eliminated from the body.[23,24] Also widely accepted is the fact that alcoholics may suffer deadly bacterial pneumonia.[25]

In recent years, alcohol, particularly the red wine, has been touted as having health benefits of reducing the risk of coronary heart disease. Such publicity has been made based on several publications.[26-29] Red wine and some alcoholic beverages have antioxidants polyphenols (the flavonols) which indeed reduce cardiovascular risks. However, the alcohol in these drinks is toxic to the brain and the liver. Since polyphenols are present in many vegetables and fruits such as grapes, drinking pure juice instead of alcoholic beverages have all the healthful properties without any of the injurious ones.[30] Cardiologist Dr. R.A. Vogel of University of Maryland stated in a review article: "Despite the wealth of observational data, it is not absolutely clear that alcohol reduces cardiovascular risk, because no randomized controlled trials have been performed. Alcohol should never be recommended to patients to reduce cardiovascular risk as a substitute for the well-proven alternatives of appropriate diet, exercise, and drugs. Alcohol remains the number three cause of preventable premature death in this country, and the risk of alcohol habituation, abuse, and adverse effects must be considered in any patient counseling."[31]

T for tobacco – one large study involving 4,462 male subjects showed that smokers had lower antibody levels and CD8 (cells patrolling viruses and cancer cells) counts.[32] During beginning periods of smoking, there may actually be a slight enhancement of the immune function (cells are more active, attempting to rid the irritant). Soon after, however, follows a suppression of T cells, natural killer cells, and phagocytes.[33,34] Passive smoking has also shown its effect on the immune system. Children of smoking parents suffer more allergies because of derangement of a type of B lymphocyte that makes IgE antibodies responsible for allergic reactions such as hay fever, asthma, and chronic sinus problem. These children are also more prone to several types of cancer.[35]

We now know that the **FAT CAT** – six factors that lower the immune function may contribute to the emergence of cancer. On the other hand, improving your lifestyle is your guarantee of protection from cancer. What if you do develop cancer, are you going to die? The answer depends on what type of treatment you choose to receive. If you learn to use the simple treatment modalities we are sharing with you in this book, you most likely will do better. If you are treated by a doctor who does not know about the importance of diet and lifestyle modification described in this book, please tactfully inform your doctor and ask him or her to be sure to include diet and lifestyle changes; better yet, you learn to incorporate this ammunition yourself. Based on our experience and observation we can assure you that when you stop doing things that may bring on cancer (to be discussed in detail in subsequent chapters), and when you strengthen your immune function, you can stop cancer!

CHAPTER 6

HEALING CANCER FROM INSIDE OUT

The title of this chapter is taken from the title of Michael Anderson's award-winning documentary film. Replete with well-researched reports, interviews, and information, this educational film is both powerful and empowering. It would make the difference between life and death, health and illness.

Michael Anderson's father suffered from stage IV malignant melanoma, which had further metastasized during treatment. With the grim prognosis of only six months to live, the doctors sent him home where he succumbed to cancer exactly six months later. Mary Harrington too was diagnosed with stage IV malignant melanoma when her doctors prescribed chemotherapy, assuring her of an additional three to six months of life. Declining chemotherapy, she chose nutritional treatment instead. Ten months later, the doctor found her to be cancer free.

Upon extensive research, Anderson discovered not only the inefficacy of conventional cancer treatment but also the side effects which actually hastened death. In the November, 1985, issue of *Scientific American*, appeared a landmark study which stated that "fourteen years after war on cancer began, chemotherapy was somewhat effective in only 2-3 percent of all cancer cases;[1] namely, Hodgkin's disease, acute lymphocytic leukemia, testicular cancer, and choriocarcinoma." Five years later, after an investigation of major medical centers treating cancer patients with chemotherapy, renowned bio-statistician Ulrich Abel of the University of Heidelberg concluded that "For most of today's common solid cancers, the ones that cause 90% of the cancer deaths each year, chemotherapy has not proven to do any good at all."[2] In 2004, oncologists in Australia reported in *Clinical Oncology* that after chemotherapy testicular cancer has a 5 year survival of 37.7%, and Hodgkin's disease 40.3%. For advanced breast and colon cancer the 5 year survival after chemotherapy is less than 2%, and for advanced melanoma and cancers of bladder, kidney, pancreas and prostate, it is zero percent.[3] In other words, with these cancers very few patients survive beyond five years after chemotherapy. Various studies from *Journal of American Medical Association, The Lancet* (a British journal) and *New England Journal of Medicine* reported that untreated patients often live longer than treated patients. Dick Richard, MD stated: "I challenge anyone to show sound evidence that advanced breast cancer patients do better or even live longer on conventional treatment than they do when left totally untreated." He concluded: "In my experience, they don't." Allen Levin, MD further declared that "Women with breast cancer are likely to die faster with chemotherapy than without it."

The documentary interviewed several physicians and institutes teaching patients to reverse cancers using diet and lifestyle changes. They show far better results than conventional treatments. In many cases, patients with advanced cancers given up by conventional treatment were able to stop the cancer and live when they resorted to diet and lifestyle changes.

John A. McDougall, MD stated: "With few exceptions, cancer is a slow growing disease; patients should have time to think about it. The problem is that doctors often make it so urgent and put patients in a situation that they have to make a decision in hours that the breast, prostate, or colon needs to cut out. The truth of matter is that the disease has been going on for ten years before they discover it, will probably go on another 10, 15, or 20 years before it kills them. Cancer is a slow growing disease and the patient should, in a sense, be patient and consider all the possibilities, and to not panic." Dr. McDougall is one of the most knowledgeable physicians dealing with lifestyle related diseases. He has written several books to educate physicians and the general public. He and his wife operate a Health and Medical Center in Santa Rosa, California. In the past several decades, they have helped and taught many thousands of patients to overcome chronic degenerative lifestyle related diseases.

Brenda Cobb, founder and director of the Living Foods Institute in Atlanta, Georgia, teaches the plant-based living foods lifestyle both at the Institute and worldwide. Twelve years ago Brenda was discovered to have cancers of breast and cervix of uterus. With her family history of breast and cervical cancer, her doctors felt the prognosis was not good. They recommended immediate surgery. They had to operate to see how extensive the tumors were. Then they'd decide if they should remove one or both breasts and do a full or partial hysterectomy. After surgery they would determine if chemotherapy and/or radiation might be needed. This scared Brenda to no end. Being a devout Christian, she felt God had a better plan for her. Brenda Cobb healed herself with the living foods and alternative treatment. In the back cover of her book *The Living Foods Lifestyle*, she says: "I got rid of tumors, allergies, gray hair, poor eyesight, arthritis, low energy, depression, acid reflux, indigestion and 75 pounds, but that was nothing compared to my great spiritual awakening. I discovered my life's purpose and a whole new reason for living. It is my privilege and joy to bring this message to the world because in my heart I know it is the truth! I am continually amazed at my students' own testimonies of healing from all types of serious diseases when they practice these simple principles." Over a decade, Brenda and her staff in the Living Foods Institute have helped terminal patients with all kinds of cancers to recover. In addition, they have seen people with "incurable" diseases including AIDS, multiple sclerosis, lupus, Parkinson's disease, who have found recovery through diet and lifestyle changes.

This is a two-part (two-hour) documentary. Part two begins with the discussion of why there has been steady increase of all types of cancer in this past century. Some believe we have more cancer today because people live longer today. The average life span 100 years ago was shorter because of early infant death. For example with two people one lived to 90 years while another died at one year; and the average of these two is 45.5 years. Another example: one lives to 90 while another lives to 70 and the average is 80. A better way to compare average life span is to compare people who lived to 65+ years. For this group of people:

In 1900 the average life span is 77 years
In 2000 the average life span is 83 years

If we compare people who lived to 85+ years:

In 1900 the average life span is 89 years
In 2000 the average life span is 91 years

People today do live a few years longer than one century ago but not that much different when one removes the great number of infant death 100 years ago.

Okinawans live a long life yet they have a low cancer rate, when they migrate to the U.S. their cancer rate becomes same as ours. So aging does not cause cancer.

Some believe the increase of cancer in recent decades is because of environmental pollution. Of course pollution does contribute to cancer but that's not the whole story. Consider again Okinawa: it's heavily industrialized and polluted but with low cancer rate. We now know only 3-5% of all cancer are caused by pollution and environmental carcinogens.

Another cause of cancer is radiation. That radiation may be harmful is indisputable. But just how harmful? John Gofman, MD, PhD has made this startling statement about the impact of medical radiation: "Our estimate is that about 75% of the current annual incidence of breast cancer in the U.S. is being caused by ionizing radiation exposure, primarily from medical sources. While medical radiation does contribute to cancer, it is not the major cause."[4]

Some blame cancer on genetics. But genetics account for only about 2-3% of all cancers. People inherit bad habits and lifestyle, not the bad genes, from parents. Today we also know that we can put bad genes to sleep by proper diet and lifestyle. My own lab actually published a paper in 1997 showing we can keep bad gene at bay by a garlic compound.[5]

Dr. Colin Campbell discusses in great length how an animal-based diet fertilizes bad genes, causing their expression, while a whole foods plant-based diet does just the opposite.[6] Nutrients indeed control gene expression.

Thomas Lodi, MD, concurs that a bad diet, not bad genes causes cancer. His clinical experiences revealed that major cancers can be cured by diet. Dr. Lodi, a graduate of University of Hawaii School of Medicine and trained in Internal Medicine, Integrative Oncology, and Metabolic Medicine, is a certified nutrition specialist, a licensed Homeopathic Physician in Arizona. He is founder and chief physician of *An Oasis of Healing*, an alternative cancer healing center in Mesa, Arizona, where many terminal and advanced stage cancer patients have reversed their diseases. The main form of treatment is a plant-based diet and green juices. Which in certain cases is supplemented with a low dose chemotherapy called Insulin Potentiation Therapy (IPT).

Adding to the conundrum of cancer causation, there are a number of interesting questions in this second part of the film:

Take for example the fact Japan leads in the consumption of cigarettes in the world and yet it boasts the lowest incidence of lung cancer. By contrast, cigarette smoking in the U.S. has dropped more than 50% in recent decades, but lung cancer continues to climb. Moreover, many lung cancer patients have never smoked. Likewise, we are witnessing an epidemic of skin cancer today when 100 years ago, people spent considerable more time outdoors than today and yet skin cancer incidence was low. These all suggest that something else is going on in our body.

Let's look at the dietary composition today as compared to 100 years ago. Below is the comparison of the percentage of calories consumed from three food sources:

	Historical percentage	Current Percentage
Animal foods	5%	42%
Refined/processed foods	0%	51%
Whole plant foods	95%	7%

The evidence is clearly linking the rise in cancer incidence with the spiraling increase in animal and refined foods coupled with the drastic decrease in whole plant foods. Dr. Campbell's studies show environmental factors are seeds for cancer, and animal foods (particularly animal protein) fertilize the cancer seeds for more abundant growth.

Can cancer be reversed by diet? Let's examine this illustration:

Cancer cell has a protein coating that is invisible to immune system. Normally our pancreas makes enzymes trypsin and chymotrypsin that can dissolve the protein coating on the surface of cancer cell so that it is visible to the immune cell to recognize it and to destroy it. With a diet high in animal protein, the pancreatic enzymes are used up to digest the dietary protein, thereby reducing the pancreatic enzymes available to digest the protein coating on the cancer cell. In contrast, pancreatic enzymes are not needed to digest vegetable protein. Regardless of the amount of vegetables eaten, the supply of pancreatic enzymes to unmask cancer cells remains plentiful. Dr. Campbell's study incontrovertibly demonstrates that animal protein promotes cancer, while vegetable protein does not. Can cancer be reversed? If so, how? The answer is simple. By greatly reducing (ideally eliminating) dietary animal protein and just eating whole plant based foods. This approach has been utilized since 1956 by probably the oldest natural health center in the U.S., the Hippocrates Health Institute in West Palm Beach, Florida. Under the leadership of Brian Clement, PhD, this Institute conducts classes teaching people how to overcome chronic degenerative diseases through nutrition and lifestyle changes.

Michael Anderson's book, also with the same title as the documentary: *Healing Cancer From Inside Out*, cites hundreds of references dealing with conventional as well as alternative treatments, particularly nutritional treatment for cancer. I have shared the documentary video with a few oncologist friends. Somewhat dubious about the effectiveness of diet and lifestyle, they nonetheless admitted to a sense of helplessness about the sustained effects of conventional cancer treatments.

My hope is that more and more professionals will take time to investigate the matter. Despite the plethora of credible scientific publications, change comes slowly. From my own clinical experiences,

I know chemotherapy and radiation do not cure cancer. They may temporarily suppress the cancer growth, but unless cancer cells are killed and immune cells simultaneously strengthened, recurrence is inevitable. As an immunologist, I concur with the doctors in the documentary who unequivocally declared that the only system that can effectively destroy cancer is the immune system. The way to nurture the immune system is through nutrition — a plant-based diet. Unfortunately, we teach very little nutritional therapy in the medical schools. My hope is my colleagues will investigate the scientific literature dealing with diet and cancer and to incorporate nutrition and lifestyle changes into their treatment protocol. And I urge you the consumer to study and to use it as well. Together we can greatly reduce the number of death caused by cancer in the U.S. and in the world.

CHAPTER 7

OBSERVATIONAL RESEARCH

This was a miserable year in my life: five of my close acquaintances (three colleagues and two close friends) were diagnosed with lung cancer. They all died in spite of chemotherapy. Four of them died within three months of undergoing the treatment. One completed the course of chemotherapy and was told that his cancer had gone into remission, but 18 months later, he had recurrence and received another round of chemotherapy. Unfortunately, before even completing this second round, he died.

During that same year, I also witnessed the death of six women, wives of colleagues and friends, who had advanced stages of breast cancer. They all had received the best surgery, radiation and chemotherapy in the nation's top medical centers. Despite the best conventional treatments, five of the women lived for only three to four years. The other woman lived for five years and four months after the initial diagnosis and treatment. Because she had passed the official five-year cancer survival marker, albeit by an additional four months, she was nonetheless considered cured and included in the cure rate statistics.

Because of my involvement in basic cancer research, I attend the annual meetings of the American Association for Cancer Research (AACR) nearly every year. One of the most exciting parts of the meetings is the reporting of new breakthroughs in cancer treatment. I began wondering why my friends and colleagues were so unfortunate in that they did not benefit from these breakthroughs. I began asking oncologists about their treatment outcomes with advanced breast and lung cancer. When queried further beyond their answers of "pretty good," most of them were unable to give me their five-year survival rates, since they themselves do not keep record. Apparently only the Medical Records Department has that information. Some of the oncologists I had befriended did say that their five-year survivals for advanced breast and lung cancers are about five percent. In other words, five out of one hundred patients so treated lived for more than five years. That is to say that 95% of the patients did not survive for five years.

Among patients in my clinic are two cancer survivors both of whom are now in their sixties. They had both been diagnosed with breast cancer more than ten years ago, but instead of conventional treatments, they chose to receive nutritional and alternative treatments from an educational center called Optimum Health Institute (OHI) in San Diego, California. They urged my wife and me to check out the program which we did. We spent a week observing and participating in educational and "how-to" classes, a wholesome plant-based diet, and detoxification through juicing and/or colon cleansing. While there, we met a dozen or so "alumni"—the cancer survivors of five to twenty years who returned for refresher courses. Incidentally, OHI does not treat any diseases, certainly not cancer. The institute is a health education center. The program aims at enhancing a person's physical, emotional, and spiritual health.

Visits to other health centers in the U.S. and abroad brought to our attention one common feature: promoting an animal-free, unprocessed, plant-based diet. As mentioned in other chapters in this book, research in recent years has consistently shown that animal products provide a triple "whammy" by 1) feeding the cancer cells, 2) protecting the cancer cells from the body's cancer-fighting immune cells, and 3) preventing the body from obtaining the nutrients it needs. Once we stop using animal products and shift to a plant-based diet, we stop feeding cancer and we start strengthening our immune cells so that they once again are ready to battle cancer. However, if the tumor or cancer is sizeable, the immune cells may not be able to fight it off, thereby requiring the additional help of conventional therapy. In Chapter 2, I mentioned when the tumor mass is large, it needs to be de-bulked by surgery, radiation, or chemotherapy. However, it is imperative to realize that these methods may not destroy all the cancer cells, which explains the recurrence of cancer after treatment. Furthermore, radiation and chemotherapy often depress the immune function.[1,2]

When I was director of the immunology research laboratory of the radiation oncology department at Loma Linda University Medical Center, my associates and I studied the immune responses of 60 patients undergoing therapeutic irradiation. We found the values of tests measuring cellular and humoral immunity were depressed during irradiation. This depression persisted until about two months after completion of treatment. By six months, the responses rose to pretreatment levels. When response was evaluated according to sites irradiated, the pelvic and pelvic plus abdominal groups showed consistently greater depression than the chest or head and neck groups. Seventeen patients who had developed metastasis or who had died from the disease had significantly greater immune depression during irradiation, suggesting that the degree of immune suppression correlates with the clinical outcome.[1] Because conventional treatments do suppress the normal immune functions, as discussed in Chapter 2 of this book, I recommend low doses of these treatments to minimize the devastating adverse side effects of such treatments. This is in opposition to conventional thinking that "more is better." We now know that the only system that can do a complete job to stop cancer growth is the immune system, our body's own defense. We now also know that animal products and refined foods intimidate the immune system while a wholesome plant-based diet strengthens it.

In the past 25 years my wife, a dietitian/nutritionist, has helped innumerable patients to recover from cancer with nutritional therapy. One 46-year-old woman had a breast tumor about the size of a walnut which was shown by biopsy to be malignant. Her doctor advised a lumpectomy to remove the tumor, followed by radiation and/or chemotherapy. She, however, chose to attend the Weimar Center of Health & Education in Northern California to participate in the NEWSTART* Lifestyle Program (www.newstart.com). NEWSTART is an acronym for eight natural remedies: N for nutrition (a plant-based diet), E for exercise, W for water (hydrotherapy), S for sun light (heliotherapy), T for temperance or moderation, A for (fresh) air, R for rest, and T for trust in divine power.

Less than a month after her stay at Weimar Center, she noticed that her lump was diminishing in size. She returned home, committed to continue the healthful living that she had learned from Weimar Center. By the end of three months, the lump was no longer detectable. This woman has since been teaching people in her church to eat a plant-based diet to stay healthy.

Another woman, 33 years of age, found a 1 x 2.5 inch breast tumor which was shown by biopsy to be malignant, as were the lymph nodes in her armpit. Her doctor wanted her to undergo mastectomy, followed by chemotherapy. Because her own mother died of breast cancer shortly after mastectomy and chemotherapy, she declined these treatments. Then six years later, she noted that the lump grown harder and a bit larger. The biopsy again showing malignant cancer. The pathology slides were examined by three pathologists and all agreed it was malignant. When she came to see us, she made it very clear that her husband and she had prayed over this matter and had again determined to decline conventional treatments. She just wanted to know if there was an alternative treatment. I ordered two blood tests for her. One is called CA 15-3, and the other Breast Carcinoma Associated Antigen 27.29. These tests detect cancer antigens in the blood. Even though few doctors use these tests, as an immunologist I have found these immunological assays to be more meaningful than the pathology slides. This woman's test results showed her readings to be very low and within normal range. To me, this meant her tumor was confined to the local site, and hence only a very low level of cancer antigen was detected in the blood. This to me was a good sign.

Since she and her husband had already decided not to receive any conventional treatment, my wife suggested that she and her husband take a vacation and spend three weeks at Optimum Health Institute in San Diego. After they completed the three week training, the whole family adopted a strict plant-based diet. Additionally, she used hydrotherapy. She felt very well and alive, but the lump changed neither in size nor hardness. After two additional years, while she maintained the wholesome plant-based diet, she continued to feel well and vibrant; but I wanted to repeat the Breast Carcinoma Associated Antigen 27.29

test. Again it was very low, within the normal range. I finally requested a plastic surgeon to remove the hard lump. The pathology report showed the lump to be not cancer, but only scar tissue (dead cells). Apparently her lifestyle changes had strengthened her defense system sufficiently to destroy the tumor. This is reminiscent of the mouse bladder tumor study we did with garlic extract, reported in Chapter 2. When we examined the group treated with garlic, the nodules turned out to be scar tissue of dead cells.

Four years ago during our last month of teaching in China, an email informed me a very close colleague had just been diagnosed with pancreatic cancer. I emailed back asking him to just sit tight not to do anything till I got back. Unfortunately the oncologist talked him into chemotherapy. When I returned from my trip, I had to attend his funeral as he died only few days after chemotherapy. I regretted that I did not have chance to help this colleague. However, meanwhile my wife was able to counsel a middle aged man with pancreatic cancer to make a complete change in his diet and lifestyle habits. He drank vegetable juices every day and the tumor gradually shrank. This man is still alive and healthy today.

Six years ago while visiting Taiwan, I was introduced to a book written in Chinese by Dr. Tom Wu, who at the age of 30, was diagnosed with advanced stage lung cancer. Modern medicine gave him no hope; it was too late to remove the damaged parts of the lung, as the cancer had already spread to other organs. His doctor predicted that he had only a few months to live. In his despair, Dr. Wu picked up the Bible and prayed. The Bible fell to the floor, whereupon he picked it up and began reading the page where it had opened. His reading was about God's creation of the earth and filling it with everything needed for human beings. Then after creating Adam and Eve, God told them that the plants, vegetables and seeded fruits growing on earth have been provided for them to eat (Genesis 1:29).

"I thought about what I had eaten in the past—meat, fish, fried and grilled food, sweet cake, but God simply wanted us to eat vegetables and fresh fruits. I was confused and doubted whether I would become weak if I ate so many vegetables and no meat," said Dr. Wu.

Yet he decided to follow the Bible's guidance. He consumed considerable amount of vegetables and fruits, clean water, and he completely adjusted his lifestyle—his sleeping, breathing, and exercise habits. Nine months later, he went for a check-up, and surprisingly no cancer cells were detected. Dr. Wu continued his new lifestyle and gets a clean bill of his health on every yearly check-up. He is now in his 70s and has been cancer free for 40 years.

Also while in Taiwan, I was introduced to three gentlemen who had been diagnosed with lung cancer by university and government hospitals. They declined conventional treatments, and instead, followed the nutritional therapy described in Dr. Wu's book. Now after more than five years, they remain alive and well. According to the five-year survival criterion used in the cancer field, these three lung cancer patients are now cured. This observation again confirms that nutrition and lifestyle changes are powerful in stopping cancer.

Five years ago during our final week teaching at the health center in China, a prominent business man brought his mother to see us. For four years she had suffered from a type of bladder cancer that does not kill quickly but does require surgery every few months because of its rapid growth pattern. This woman had endured five surgeries already, and we found her tumor to be about the size of an orange. She informed us that her diet was considered the best – expensive rich foods. Fruits and vegetables, she claimed, were for poor people. At the center, the young doctor changed her diet and incorporated hydrotherapy into her treatment plan. A month after we returned to the U.S., the doctor called to inform us that her bladder tumor had shrunk to half its size, and a few months later, the tumor had completely disappeared. Her son was so happy with such an outcome that he opened a vegan restaurant in the city expose people to the benefits of a healthy diet and lifestyle.

This reminds me of the two patients with colon cancer we saw in our clinic a few years ago. Both of them (one male and one female) opted to use a plant-based diet instead of conventional treatment. They reported that tumors fell off by themselves (six months in one and eight months in the other). These cases are examples of non-surgical surgery we referred to elsewhere in this book, meaning a plant-based diet can cause the cancer/tumor to fall off without a scalpel.

I had opportunity to investigate the nutritional therapy for cancer carried out by Phillip E. Binzel, Jr., MD. He reported the results of cancer patients he treated over a period of 18 years from 1974 through the end of 1991.[3] All of these patients were diagnosed by other physicians and the diagnoses were confirmed by pathology reports. Dr. Binzel divided his cancer patients into two groups. The first group included those with the primary cancer, meaning cancer confined to a single area with perhaps a few adjacent lymph nodes involved. The second group is known as the metastatic cancer that included those whose primary cancer had spread into other distant area of the body. Of the primary cancer group, there were 180 patients with 30 different types of cancer. Over a period of 18 years, 35 died of cancer while seven died of other causes. One hundred and thirty-eight of these patients were alive in 1991 when he wrote the report. Fifty-eight of these patients (42%) had a follow-up of between two years and four years. Eighty of these patients (58%) had a follow-up of between five and eighteen years, as compared to only 15% five-year survival rate of those with primary cancer with early diagnosis and early treatment (surgery and/or radiation and/or chemotherapy), based on the American Cancer Society statistics. In this case, nutritional therapy indeed did better than the conventional treatments.

With the metastatic group, there were 108 patients representing 23 different types of cancer. Again, the diagnoses were made by other physicians with confirmation by pathologists. From the period 1974 through 1991 a total of 47 patients died: thirty-two of the patients died from their disease, six died of causes unrelated to their disease, and nine died of causes unknown. Sixty-one patients were well and alive at the time of his report. Thirty of them (49%) had a follow-up of between two and four years while 31 of them (51%) had a follow-up of between five and eighteen years. By contrast, the American Cancer Society statistics show that in metastatic disease, the conventional treatments have a five-year survival rate of only 0.1%, or one in one thousand (as compared to 51% in Dr. Binzel's group). Again, in this case, nutritional therapy outcomes incontrovertibly superseded that of the conventional therapy.

Similar to other centers using nutritional therapy, Dr. Binzel's program emphasizes a plant-based diet with avoidance of animal products and refined sugars. Dr. Binzel also uses Laetrile (vitamin B17), a proprietary product rich in nitriloside. The enzyme beta-glucosidase produced by intestinal bacteria can break down nitriloside to yield molecules of glucose, benzaldehyde, and hydrogen cyanide. Both hydrogen cyanide and benzaldehyde are toxic to mammalian cells. However, in human body hydrogen cyanide is readily converted to non-toxic thiocyanate by enzyme rhodanese (thiosulfate transulfurase) while benzaldehyde is being oxidized to harmless benzoic acid. So under normal condition nitriloside is not toxic to human body. Instead, the normal metabolism of nitriloside actually provides additional nutrients for the body cells. It is a different story when nitriloside encounters cancer cells. The enzyme beta-glucosidase in cancer cells also breaks down nitriloside to yield molecules of glucose, benzaldehyde, and hydrogen cyanide. The difference is: cancer cells do not utilize an oxidative metabolic pathway; instead, it uses a fermentative or anaerobic pathway (this was discovered by Nobel Prize laureate Otto Warburg, a prominent German chemist long ago). Because of this, benzaldehyde is not oxidized to non-toxic benzoic acid in cancer cells. Furthermore, cancer cells also lack the enzyme rhodanese and hence cannot convert hydrogen cyanide to non-toxic thiocyanate. Nitriloside thus shows selective toxicity to cancer cells. Incidentally, nitriloside or Laetrile has been a very controversial subject. The FDA (Food and Drug Administration) prohibits its use in the U.S. Since nitriloside is found in many plants, in the kernels of seeds of fruits, some vegetables, and in beans and grains, which are actually seeds. A plant-based diet thus provides ample supply of nitriloside. It is, therefore, no need to use Laetrile and accrue additional expense. Simply eat the fruits/vegetables with their seeds, and also eat beans and grains.

I would like to conduct one more observational research. Call it survey type of research if you like. In fact, I would like to invite you to do this survey type of research together with me. I'll give you the instruction as how to do it. We will get the data from the organization called Hallelujah Acres founded by Dr. George Malkmus. (In 1976, at the age of 42, Dr. Malkmus, a dynamic Baptist minister, was diagnosed with colon cancer. This diagnosis was made only a short time after he had watched his mother die as a result of cancer following several years of medical treatments. Her illness and deterioration was a terrible thing to have to witness. Dr. Malkmus believed that his mother suffered more from the treatments she received than she did from the cancer itself. After watching his mother go through this terrible ordeal, he determined to find alternative treatment for cancer. After extensive researching, he made changes in his nutrition and lifestyle, and within a year, he was completely well, not only from cancer but also from other health problems he had before.[4] Today, 35 years later, Dr. Malkmus continues to enjoy excellent health. In the past 30 plus years, he has been conducting health seminars teaching people all over the world how to live a healthy life free from disease. His educational program is based on biblical teachings). Sorry, for such a long footnote.

Back to the research we're going to do together. For this you need a computer with the internet service. Here are the steps:

1. Turn on the computer and the internet. Go to the home page of Hallelujah Acres. Or use any search engine (Yahoo, Google, etc.) type in www.hacres.com.

2. When you see the home page of Hallelujah Acres, on the top tool bar click Testimonies.

3. Scroll down the page you will find Testimony Data Base in alphabetical order: Allergies (90), Arthritis (163), Asthma (81), Back pain (59), Blood pressure and cholesterol (193), Bone (16), Cancer (280), etc. There are many more. As you can see this is a large data base. We are interested in Cancer (280). The number in the brackets refers to the number of cases.

4. We can read all the 280 testimonies sent to Hallelujah Acres center voluntarily by individuals (cancer survivors) who have benefited from doing two important things: One, stopping the consumption of all animal products and processed foods; and Two, adopting a wholesome plant-based diet. Sixty five women have overcome breast cancer. Among them are those

who had surgery, radiation, and chemotherapy but did not stop the cancer from growing. On dying bed, as a last resort, they adopted the plant-based diet. They wrote to testify that they are now cancer free. Some women did not have conventional treatment but chose to use nutrition to fight their breast cancer. These individuals witness healing of cancer; even faster than those already had other forms of treatment.

5.   There are twenty-six cases of prostate cancer recovered with the plant-based nutrition, including some very advanced terminal cases that conventional therapists had nothing more to offer— they were told to go home to take care of their affairs. Obviously they were ecstatic to have their lives back with a plant-based nutrition.

6.   There are survivors of 13 cases of colon cancer, 8 cases of ovarian cancer, and 7 cases of lung cancer. In addition, plant-based diet also helped individuals with bladder cancer, kidney cancer, liver cancer, stomach cancer, pancreatic cancer, etc.

This is a research I want you to do it together with me. If you do not have time to read all 280 testimonies, you can choose whatever cases you would like to read. Then see if your conclusion agrees with mine. The conclusion I draw from this observation is that plant-based nutritional therapy (phytotherapy) is simple, yet exceedingly powerful.

Elsewhere in this book, we note that animal products and processed foods, particularly refined sugars, feed cancer cells. Once these foods are removed from our diet, cancer cells stop further growth. Elimination of such foods also removes the protective protein coating on cancer cell surfaces so that the immune cells are once again able to recognize and kill off the cancer cells. Replacing the deleterious animal products and processed foods with wholesome plant foods strengthens the immune cells so that they once again are ready to destroy the cancer cells. The simplicity of a plant-based diet disguises its powerful effectiveness. It in essence provides three types of therapies: Phytotherapy is a type of 1) immunotherapy, 2) non-surgical surgery, and 3) chemotherapy without the adverse side effects.

CHAPTER 8

TOXIC ENVIRONMENT

In Chapter 2, we learned that cancer is caused by chemical carcinogens, radiation, and viruses. However, other factors may contribute to cancer development. In the next three chapters we will consider the toxic environment, toxic lifestyle habits, and the toxic diet on the development of cancer in the human body, and ways to minimize them.

Let's look at toxic environment. Dr. T. Colin Campbell, noted authority in nutrition says that cancer is largely "due to environmental/lifestyle factors, and not genetics."[1] We are living in the most toxic environment in the history of humankind. More than 4 billion pounds of toxic chemicals were released into the environment in 2011. Most of these chemicals were found in the ground and in the water.[2] Partial list of the potential carcinogenic compounds are found in our environment include:

- Pesticides/herbicides and other toxic chemicals
- Chlorine byproducts
- Asbestos
- Fiberglass
- Nuclear-radiation

Pesticides, Herbicides and Other Toxic Chemicals

All of us – even newborns are daily exposed to pesticides, herbicides and other toxic chemicals. These chemicals are found in agriculture crop, household and garden products, surface and ground water. Toxic chemicals are also found in animal foods.

Pesticides: One of the most commonly-used pesticides is the organophosphates. The U.S. Environmental Protection Agency lists the organophosphate parathion as a possible carcinogen.[3] Many pesticides produce estrogenic effects that mimic estrogens in our bodies, which in turn may contribute to hormone-related cancers such as cancers of the breast, uterus, ovaries, and prostate.[4]

Even before birth, the fetus already harbors toxins. Laboratory tests have detected Bisphenol A (BPA), a plastic component and synthetic estrogen, in umbilical cord blood of infants in the United States.[5] This chemical crosses the placenta barrier, producing defects in the offspring.[6] Particularly alarming is the fact that toxic chemicals, often stored in the body fat cells, can be passed on for generations.

The incidence of childhood leukemia and brain cancer continues to climb. It is disheartening to realize that testicular cancer among young men in the 15-30 year-old bracket has jumped by more than 50 percent.[7]

Plastics: Phthalates are a group of chemicals found in many plastic products. The chemicals can enter our bodies through food, air, and skin. Exposure to phthalates is often through food during processing and storage; and may also occur during medical procedures. Phthalates are classified as "probable human carcinogens," causing a wide range of adverse health problems.[8]

The Centers for Disease Control have identified 148 toxic chemicals in the blood and urine of people of all ages in the United States.[9] Scientists have detected urinary levels of phthalate metabolites in over 75 percent of the samples collected – with children having significantly higher levels than adults.[10]

Food: Consumption of animal foods including milk and dairy products is another source of toxic chemicals. Due to animal diseases and the need to increase production for profit, animals are routinely given antibiotics, growth hormones, steroids and drugs. In addition, these animals are also exposed to pesticides, herbicides, and toxic chemicals. Certain chemicals contain carcinogens have caused hundreds of deaths among the factory farm livestock.[11,12]

Researchers also noted that large fish in Lake Michigan and the Great Lakes area are contaminated with polychlorinated biphenyls (PCBs), mercury, and other chemicals. Adults who drink water containing

PCBs could experience immune deficiencies, thymus, reproductive, and nervous system disorders along with an increased risk of cancer.[13]

Animal consumption in the United States exceeds that of other countries. Our annual meat consumption tops at 275 pounds per person follow with Spain at 261 pounds, India at 11 pounds and Bangladesh at 6.8 pounds per person.[14] Each year nearly 10 billion land animals are slaughtered for food.[15] More than 9 billion of just chicken alone, are consumed annually.[16]

Chlorine Byproducts

Chlorine has been used to treat public water supplies. But when combined with other chemicals, chlorine produces byproducts which are extremely toxic which over time can cause immune system breakdown.[17]

Dioxin: Of all the man-made chemicals known to science, dioxin is considered the most carcinogenic. A chlorine byproduct increases the risk of liver and lung cancer, dioxin also interferes with the immune system resulting in a higher risk of infectious diseases. Dioxins are formed as byproducts in industrial and combustion processes. These chemicals then enter streams and waterways where they are absorbed by fish and agricultural crops. Eventually the toxic chemicals can go up the food chain to livestock and poultry. Dioxin is found in the highest concentration in foods that are high in animal fat, such as milk, dairy products, meat, fish, and eggs.[18]

Asbestos

Asbestos has been classified as a known human carcinogen. In spite of the sharp decline in asbestos use, the incidence of asbestos-related disease continues to rise. The time between exposure to asbestos and the development of cancer may take 10 to 40 years or more after exposure for asbestos-related symptoms to appear.[19]

Study showed that naturally occurring asbestos significantly elevate the mortality rates of nasopharyngeal and laryngeal cancer, intestinal cancer, lung cancer, and mesothelioma. This may be due to changes in the land distribution. With higher proportions of farmland and urban area; and lower proportions of forested land have contributed to an increase in the mortality rate of these cancers.[20]

Fiberglass

Fiberglass may also be carcinogenic. It is found in nearly every building and home. Studies conducted by the National Cancer Institute reported that glass fibers were potent carcinogens in both experimental animals and humans.[21] Occupational exposures to glass fibers, mineral wood fibers, and brick dust showed significant associations with increased risk of renal cell carcinoma.[22]

Nuclear Radiation

Nuclear radiation is becoming more widespread than ever before. It appears that there is a correlation between exposure and higher incidence of cancers such as, thyroid, bone marrow (white blood cells), breast, and lung.[23]

Radiation damage to our DNA is cumulative over a lifetime.[24] With the advancement in technology, and the extensive use of electronic appliances, gadgets, and microwave ovens, our exposure to radiation is escalating. Although a causal relationship remains inconclusive, minimizing exposure nevertheless remains a prudent choice.

How can we reduce our exposure to toxic chemicals?

One of the most effective ways is to eliminate or at least greatly reduce our consumption of animal foods. The reason – over 90 per cent of toxic chemicals come from animal foods and less than 10 per cent come from plant foods.[25]

What about organic meat and animal products – aren't they safer? Unfortunately, even organically raised animals very likely also harbor toxins within their bodies from the environment, water, and animal feed which may contain agricultural herbicides/pesticides. We know that toxic chemicals tend to concentrate in the fatty tissues of animals much more than in fruits and vegetables. In other words, animal foods contain more toxic chemicals because animals bio-accumulate and, thereby, bio-intensify the cancer-causing chemicals in their body-fat, which are then passed on to us when we eat them. A noted pesticide authority Lewis Regenstein stated that "Meat contains approximately 14 times more pesticides than do plant foods; dairy products 5 1/2 times more. Thus, by eating foods of animal origin, one ingests greatly concentrated amounts of toxic chemicals. Analysis of various foods by the FDA shows that meat, poultry, fish, cheese and other dairy products contain levels of these pesticides more often and in greater amount than other foods."[26]

Remember that a healthy immune system is vital for destroying cancer cells. Daily exposure to environmental toxins weakens our immunity. We need to minimize our exposure and keep our immune function at its peak. Here are some ways to protect ourselves:

1. Eliminate or greatly reduce consumption of animal foods, eggs, milk, and dairy products.
2. Avoid the use of toxic chemicals found in household cleaning products, garden pesticides, and personal care products.
3. Use filtered drinking water.
4. Use organically grown produce whenever possible.
5. Store food items in glass, ceramic, or stainless steel containers. Avoid or greatly reduce the use of plastic for food storage.
6. Avoid or greatly minimize microwave cooking.

CHAPTER 9

TOXIC LIFESTYLE HABITS

Cancer is largely a preventable disease that is lifestyle-dependent. Most cancers are caused by what we eat and how we live.[1,2] In this chapter, we will consider certain lifestyle habits that may damage our immune system and greatly increase our cancer risks.

Tobacco: Smoking harms nearly every organ of the body – causing approximately 30 percent of all cancer deaths in the United States. In addition to lung cancer, smoking has been linked to leukemia and other cancers, such as cancer of the head, neck, mouth, throat, vocal cords, bladder, kidney, stomach, cervix, and pancreas.[3]

Alcohol: Alcohol, a leading preventable cause of cancer deaths in this country, is a known carcinogen even when consumed in *small quantities*. Boston University School of Medicine found that 30 percent of the reported deaths from alcoholism were by those who consumed 1.5 drinks or less a day, raising the possibility that no amount of alcohol is safe. Breast cancer was the most common drinking-related deaths in women.[4] For men, mouth, throat, and esophageal cancers are the most common alcohol-associated deaths.[4] The risk for cancers of the liver, colon, and rectum are also increased with alcohol consumption. Alcoholic beverages contain sugar which feeds cancer. Sugar along with the alcohol-induced new blood vessel growth, promotes even greater proliferation of cancer cells.[5]

Synthetic Hormones: The use of synthetic hormones by women remains controversial. Research shows that synthetic estrogen stimulates cell growth and increases cancer risk. It also inhibits apoptosis in estrogen receptor-positive breast cancer cells.[6] Apoptosis refers to the normal process of programmed cell deaths. Rather than dying, cancer cells continue multiplying and dividing. High levels of estrogen, known as "estrogen dominance" are associated with many health problems. One of the most common causes of estrogen dominance is a class of compounds known as *xenoestrogens,* which are man-made compounds. These are foreign estrogens that mimic the effects of natural estrogens. They act like "hormone disruptors" that wreak havoc in the body.[7] Xenoestrogens are found in non-organic produce that have been sprayed with pesticides and other chemicals; as well as in meat and dairy products. Estrogens are fed to dairy cattle to encourage milk production and to chickens to increase egg production. Refined and processed foods also contain toxic additives. Furthermore, inadequate consumption of protective phytonutrients found in organic fresh fruits and vegetables raises the risk of cancer as well.[8]

To protect against xenoestrogens, we need to:

1. Avoid using insecticides, pesticides, and household chemicals.
2. Avoid eating animal foods, and dairy products.
3. Avoid eating processed foods with preservatives and chemicals which are xenoestrogenic.
4. Reduce the use of plastic products, and avoid chemicals in personal care products.[9]

Medical and Dental X-rays: CBS evening news reported that Americans waste $700 billion each year on unnecessary medical tests. Health care constitutes 17% of the entire U.S. economy, one-third of which is spent on unnecessary tests. In our litigious society, physicians practice defensive medicine by ordering more tests than necessary. A potential danger of excessive medical screenings is the increased exposure to radiation and procedures of which the benefits may not outweigh the risks.

Radiation is an inescapable part of life. In addition to exposure to ionizing radiation from natural sources, such as from the soil and sun, we also get radiation from X-rays, and nuclear-power plants.[10] Avoiding unnecessary exposure is nothing short of prudence.

Chronic Stress: Stress is an inevitable part of life, but chronic stress can raise cancer risk and weaken our immune system. A weakened immunity leads to tumors. Several animal studies have confirmed such effects.[11,12,13] On the other hand, stress per se is not the culprit. Rather, it is the "persistent perception of helplessness" that is damaging.[14]

Despite the inevitability of stress in our daily lives, our attitude can effectively help us cope. Rather than remaining locked in a victimized state of "helplessness," we can change our attitude. A Biblical injunction tells us to "Be thankful, whatever the circumstances may be." (1 Thessalonians 5:18, Phillips translation). While some factors in life are beyond our control, our attitude is one element of our life that is under our control and our control alone. An attitude of gratitude can make a great difference in our physical, emotional, and spiritual health.

Prescription Drugs: We know all drugs have adverse side effects, and some prescribed medications are linked to increased cancer risk. The Institute for Safe Medication Practices reported that nearly 142,000 serious, disabling or fatal adverse drug events occur each year; and such adverse effects are on the rise.[15]

How effective are cancer treatments?

A clear cut answer remains debatable. A study conducted at the Fred Hutchinson Cancer Research Center in Seattle found evidence of DNA damage in the healthy cells after chemotherapy treatment. The scientists noted that these damaged cells secreted more of a protein which boosts cancer cell survival. That is, they interact with nearby tumor cells and *cause them to grow, invade, and resist subsequent therapy.* The study showed that chemotherapy can damage DNA, promote tumor cell survival, and disease progression.[16] Research has also indicated that tumor/cancer often responds well initially, which then is followed by rapid regrowth, and finally by resistance to further treatments. Simply put: chemotherapy can *extend cancer cell survival, cause cancer to spread, and enhance subsequent treatment resistance.*

Until we remove the toxic lifestyle habits, a cure for cancer may remain elusive because any sustainable cure requires a strong immune system supported by wholesome foods and healthy lifestyle habits.

CHAPTER 10

TOXIC DIET

Cancer does not randomly strike. *Our toxic diet is the most important contributory factor for cancer.*[1,2] Daily food choices play a prominent role in the rise of cancer incidences and deaths. The National Research Council reports that diet is the greatest single factor in the epidemic of cancers of the breast, colon, and prostate. Other types of cancer are also linked to certain foods.[2] In fact improper diet causes more cancer deaths every year than cigarette smoking. Being obese or smoking more than 10 cigarettes a day doubles the death risks.[3]

What Type of Diet is Linked to Cancer?

Our typical Western diet, abundant in animal foods, high in fats and sugars, loaded with toxins, and highly processed, contributes to cancer. These foods are cancer promoters. Today's diet contains a minimal amount of protective phytochemicals which are cancer fighters.[4] Sadly, our Western diet may be the fertilizer of a cancer-prone population. Take a look at how our current diet promotes cancer:

Today's diet *feeds* cancer cells.
Today's diet *starves* normal cells.
Today's diet *weakens* immune functions.

Could this be one of the reasons that the U.S. now ranks 36th for life expectancy among 191 nations in the world? In terms of health care spending per capita, U.S. is number one, but we now rank number 37th in the assessment of health care systems.[5] How is it that we spend so much yet get so little?

Investing wisely of our resources of time, effort, and money is essential for lasting dividends. However, lifelong patterns are difficult to change and seem daunting and discouragingly arduous. Popping a pill is easier than changing our unhealthy lifestyle. No wonder we swallow pills to go sleep, to wake up, to ease pain, to control blood pressure, to lower cholesterol, to lift mood, and to calm anxiety. Yet, it behooves us to consider the ultimate consequences of our choices. First, recognize that cancer has *three mouths*!

The Three Mouths of Cancer

This was first brought to my attention when I was teaching a nutrition class in China several years ago. My students were assigned different topics to present. One young man chose "cancer and diet." For his visual aid, he plopped down a huge coconut in front of the class. At the top of the coconut protruded three straws, each pointing in a different direction. Before uttering a word, with a dramatic tilt of his head, he made an obtrusively loud slurping sound as he simultaneously tried to suck on all three straws! The whole class burst out laughing. I wondered... what was he trying to prove?

The student then wrote the Chinese character for cancer with large pictorial strokes on the white board. By so doing, he pinpointed the true culprit for this dreadful disease. You see, long ago the Chinese recognized the close link between what we eat and our health. For example, an often repeated Chinese idiom states, "Diseases come in through the mouth (what we eat), and disasters go out through the mouth" (what we say).

The Chinese character for cancer 癌 illustrates the close association between diet and disease. This word 癌 comprises three parts: 1) the Chinese character for "disease" can be found in the top short stroke and horizontal line that then goes into a downward vertical slope on the left with two short strokes, 2) "three mouths" are depicted by three squares in the inner portion of the character, and 3) the word "mountain" is characterized by the horizontal line at the bottom with its three legs sprouting upward. Thus cancer 癌 can be viewed as **disease** resulting from **three mouth**s consuming a **mountain** of food! Yes, cancer does have *three mouths!*

Cancer has a favorite food for each of its three mouths. The following is a list of cancer's three favorite cancer-producing foods:

1. Animal foods
2. Refined sugars and synthetic sweeteners
3. Refined processed grains and legumes, fats and oils

Animal Foods – Cancer's First Mouth

Animal foods are cancer promoters. Besides meat, poultry, fish, seafood, this group also includes milk, dairy, and eggs. In the United States, we consume inordinate amounts of animal products. Take chicken for example, each year we kill over 9 billion chickens for food consumption.[6] This translates to over one million chickens per hour! What components in animal foods contribute to cancer?

1. Animal protein and animal fat
2. Toxic chemicals and synthetic hormones
3. Lack of fiber
4. Cooking temperature and cooking time

Animal protein and animal fat: High intake of animal protein has been shown to increase the risk of the cancers of breast, colon, rectum, pancreas, uterus, and prostate by fueling tumor growth.[2,7,8] Generally foods high in protein are also high in fat. But when fat is removed, the protein concentration actually increases, which may also raise the cancer risk. How does animal protein favor the development of cancer?

1. *Animal protein enhances production of insulin-like growth factor (IGF-1).* Cholesterol is a predictor of heart disease. The growth hormone, Insulin-like Growth Factor (IGF-1) is a predictor of

cancer. When we eat animal-based foods, our body makes more IGF-1.[9,10] In other words, the more animal foods eaten, the more IGF-1 production, and the more cancer growth. For example, by measuring the circulating blood levels of IGF-1, researchers can predict the risk of developing advanced prostate cancer.[11]

2. *Animal protein is associated with excess insulin in diabetes.* People who eat more animal-based foods tend to develop diabetes. Excess insulin produced in diabetes can stimulate the growth of cancer cells and thereby increase the risk of cancers of the liver, pancreas, kidney, colon, stomach, and ovaries.[12]

3. *The amount of animal protein can affect cancer development.* One can turn "on" and turn "off" cancer by increasing and decreasing the quantity of protein eaten.[9] More animal protein turns "on" cancer. Less animal protein turns "off" cancer.[13] Delving deeper, we discovered those eating only plant-based foods showed a lower mean serum insulin-like growth factor-1 than those eating animal-based foods.[14] When we decrease animal food consumption, we lower the production of IGF-1 and reduce the cancer growth.

Toxic chemicals and synthetic hormones: Besides animal protein and fat, animal foods also contain toxic chemicals and synthetic hormones which are routinely given to farm animals. Cows are injected with genetically engineered growth hormones to increase milk production. The genetically altered milk has 10-20 times the IGF-1 (Insulin-like growth factor-1) levels when compared with natural cow's milk. Drinking the IGF-1-laden milk poses a greater risk for breast cancer, ovarian cancer, prostate cancer in men, and colon cancer in both men and women.[15,16]

Lack of fiber: Another reason why animal foods contribute to cancer is that they contain zero fiber. A person consuming mostly animal and refined food does not get adequate fiber which can be a factor in the development of colon cancer. The Centers for Disease Control indicate that more than 50,000 Americans die of colorectal cancer every year.[17] Dietary fiber protects against not only colorectal cancer but also cancers in the small intestines[18] and decreases the risk of breast cancer in postmenopausal women.[19]

Cooking temperature and cooking time: Higher cooking temperature and longer cooking time increase cancer risks. When meat protein is cooked at high temperatures, carcinogenic chemicals known as heterocyclic amines (HCAs) are formed. They are some of the most potent mutagens that can induce tumors in animals and increase the risk of human cancers.[20]

Using duck meat, scientists analyzed the various cooking methods on the formation of heterocyclic amines (HCAs). Pan-fried duck breast contained the highest amount of total HCAs, followed by charcoal-grilling, deep-fat-frying, roasting, microwave cooking, and boiling.[21]

Broiled and barbecued meats – Dry searing heat produces high levels of heterocyclic amines known to damage DNA. Broiling may produce 50 times as many potential carcinogens as boiling or baking. These chemicals have been linked to cancers of the colon, pancreas, breast, and prostate.[22]

Fried foods – Frying also creates carcinogens. When vegetable oils are heated, they become oxidized and yield free radicals that damage our DNA, which can then lead to cancer. High fat diets have been implicated in colon, breast, and prostate cancers.[23]

Grilled chicken - Grilled chicken products contain carcinogen called PhIP. Even in small amounts as in a grilled-chicken salad, PhIP can increase cancer risk of developing breast or prostate cancer.[24]

Animal protein and fat, plus toxic chemicals and hormones, devoid of fiber, with longer cooking time and higher temperature all contribute to cancer risks when one consumes animal-based foods.

Risks of Common Cancers from Animal-based Foods: In this section, we will look at research data regarding the relationship between consumption of animal-based foods and the risks of common cancers (breast, colon, prostate, ovarian, and pancreatic cancer).

Breast Cancer: Research has shown that animal estrogens and high fat foods increase the risk of breast cancer. Approximately three-quarters of breast cancers are fueled by estrogen. Countries that consume higher fat intake from animal products have a higher incidence of breast cancer.[25]

Red meat – The Harvard Medical School researchers found that higher consumption of red meat was strongly related to elevated risk of breast cancers. Those who ate one or more servings per day had nearly twice the risk for developing breast cancer compared with those who consumed three servings or less of red meat per week.[26] Red meat is also high in heme iron which fuels estrogen-dependent tumor growth.

Milk and cheese – As noted earlier, protein in cow's milk is "an exceptionally potent cancer promoter."[9] Those consuming cow's milk have more IGF-1, and those consuming genetically altered milk show even more IGF-1 in the bloodstream. These individuals are at higher risk for breast cancer.[27,28] Dairy consumption is associated in premenopausal breast cancer,[29] particularly with such high-fat dairy products as ice cream, cheese, and butter.[30] Surprisingly, low-fat dairy products also increases the risk for premenopausal breast cancer. Similar results were found among the Japanese. Those who consumed more meat, eggs, butter, and cheese showed greater risk of developing breast cancer.[31]

Chicken – Chicken and poultry consumption is associated with breast cancer. The carcinogen (PhIP) in grilled chicken is a potent breast cancer promoter. Our rich Western diet contains an abundance of these carcinogenic compounds.[23] Since 2005, the federal government officially added PhIP and other heterocyclic amines (HCAs) to its list of carcinogens.[32]

Colon Cancer: Americans lead the world in colon diseases and colon cancer. Current data point to the consumption of dietary fat, red meat, processed meat, dairy, and to the deficiency of nutrients as the offenders in increasing the risk of colorectal cancer.[33]

Animal-based foods and processed meats – To reduce the risk of colorectal cancer one needs to avoid animal foods, processed meat, alcohol, obesity, and also to increase daily physical activity.[34] By so doing, one can reduce the risks of many other cancers as well.[35,36,37] Just one ounce of processed meat per day increases the risk of stomach cancer by 15 to 38 percent.[38] Nitrites or nitrates are added to meats as preservatives and coloring/flavoring agents. The nitrites produce N-nitroso compounds which are carcinogens.

All animal foods promote colon cancer, yet in 1976, John Morgan, president of California's Riverside Meat Packers, proclaimed: "Beef is the backbone of the American diet.... To think that meat of all things causes cancer is ridiculous." Six years later, Mr. Morgan died of colon cancer.[39] In 2004, Charlie Bell, CEO of McDonald's fast-foods restaurants, also died from colon cancer. He was only 44. Mr. Bell began working at McDonald's at age 15 and worked there for 29 years until his untimely death.

Eggs – Eggs have been shown to be significantly correlated with mortality from colon and rectal cancers in both men and women.[40] Those who consume one and a half egg per week had five times more colorectal cancer risk than those consuming less than eleven eggs per year.[41] Most commercially prepared entrees, baked products, soups, dressings, and mixes contain both dairy and eggs.

Prostate Cancer: One man in six will be diagnosed with prostate cancer. Approximately 240,000 men will be diagnosed with prostate cancer each year.[42]

Meat, milk, dairy products, poultry, and eggs – Research data indicate that those who consume these foods have 3.6 times the incidence of prostate cancer when compared with those who ate these foods infrequently or not at all.[43] The effects of egg consumption was especially noticeable. Researchers reported that men consuming just 2.5 eggs per week increased their risk for advance prostate cancer by 81 percent compared with those who eat less than half an egg per week. Red meat, processed meat, and poultry also increase the risk of developing lethal form of prostate cancer.[44] Interestingly, cow's milk is shown to stimulate growth of prostate cancer cells by over 30 percent; while almond milk *suppressed* the growth of these cancer cells by over 30 percent.[45]

High cholesterol – A significant association has been observed between hypercholesterolemia (high cholesterol) and prostate cancer. Men with high cholesterol levels are more likely to develop prostate cancer.[46]

Dairy calcium and calcium supplements – Studies have shown that calcium intake from both supplements and dairy products increase the risk of prostate cancer.[47] Even with low-fat milk, the prostate cancer risk was elevated suggesting that dairy calcium is a potential threat to prostate health.[48,49] Interestingly, the lower prostate cancer rates among Asians swing upward when they migrate to Western countries as their diet takes on more animal-based food.[50]

Ovarian Cancer: Ovarian cancer is the deadliest gynecologic cancer in the United States. All animal products are risk factors for ovarian cancer; and the risk declines with increasing consumption of vegetables and fruits.[51,52]

Eggs – Egg consumption is associated with an increased risk of ovarian cancer, whereas eating green leafy vegetables is strongly associated with a decreased risk.[53]

Milk and dairy products – Research has shown that milk and dairy products are linked to ovarian cancer.[54] Women who drink more than one glass of milk per day had a 73 percent greater chance of getting ovarian cancer than those who drink less than one cup a day.[53] Lactose (milk sugar) can also increase the risk for ovarian cancer. When women were given yogurt to eat, investigators found that there was a highly significant trend in increased ovarian cancer risk.[55]

Refined sugar – In a population-based case-control study, the researchers found an increased risk of ovarian cancer associated with the intake of sugary drinks.[56]

Pancreatic Cancer: Animal foods, eggs, fatty foods, coffee, and sugar have all been implicated in increasing the risk of pancreatic cancer.[57] For example, when subjects ate approximately 50 grams (one sausage or 4-5 slices of bacon) every day researchers found an increased risk of 19 percent.[58] In contrast, raw fruits and vegetables have been associated with decreased risk.

Animal Foods Lead to Cancer because they are:

1. Acidic
2. High in cholesterol and fat
3. Pro-inflammatory
4. High in synthetic hormones
5. Loaded with toxic chemicals
6. Devoid of fiber
7. Devoid of protective phytonutrients

As noted in the foregoing, we can close cancer's "first mouth," which is animal food, by drastically reducing, better yet totally eliminating animal foods from our diet. All animal foods are cancer promoters. When we stop eating them, we immediately halt the camouflage process so that our powerful immune cells can once again recognize and destroy the cancer cells (Chapter 1).

Refined Sugar and Synthetic Sweeteners – Cancer's Second Mouth

Cancer's second mouth loves sweets! Refined sugars and synthetic sweeteners are also cancer promoters. How do sweets contribute to cancer development?

1. Sugar feeds cancer
2. Sugar weakens immune system by lowering our ability to fight infections
3. Sugar is a toxic chemical

The average American consumes approximately 150 to 175 pounds of sugar per year as compared to 5 pounds per year 200 years ago, a 35-fold difference! We are paying dearly for this dramatic surge. We are becoming a nation of sugar addicts. It is estimated that half of the population drink at least one sugary-drink per day. Seventy percent of teenagers drink an average of four cans of sodas per day. Women drinking two or more drinks per day are nearly four times as likely to develop high triglycerides, impair fasting glucose levels, and increase their waist girth – all risk factors for cancer.[59] Historically, this was not so. Can you believe that 200 years ago, sugar was a prescription item? Cardiovascular diseases and cancer were almost unknown back then.

Sugar is hidden in most commercially prepared foods and beverages. Some foods that may not taste sweet nonetheless contain substantial amounts of refined sugar. For example, an 8-ounce nonfat fruit yogurt has 8-10 teaspoons of sugar; a 12-ounce can soda has 10 teaspoons of sugar; white bread contains roughly 2 teaspoons sugar per slice; half a cup of spaghetti sauce has about 3 teaspoons of sugar; and even a stick of chewing gum has ½ teaspoon of sugar.

What is wrong with refined sugar? During the milling process, all valuable vitamins, minerals, enzymes, fibers, and other naturally occurring nutrients are removed. Then chemicals and bleaching solutions are added. Thus, a wholesome sugar cane is stripped of its nutrients and is turned into a toxic chemical.

The perils of refined sugar have been known for years. Now we are aware of its adverse effects on cancer. Worse yet, refined sugar actually fuels cancer.

How does sugar feed cancer? Blood glucose rises rapidly when we eat refined sugar, white flour, white rice, and numerous products made from refined grains and legumes. When blood glucose rises, it triggers the release of insulin and insulin-like growth factor (IGF-1) that stimulates cell growth and promotes inflammation. Together, insulin and IGF-1 can stimulate abnormal cell growth. The combined activities of sugar, insulin, and IGF-1 act in concert to fertilize cancer growth.[60] Then continuing their destruction, they invade neighboring tissues which results in metastasis.[61]

What about high-fructose corn syrup? High-fructose corn syrup has been linked to obesity, metabolic syndrome, diabetes, and cancer.[62] Studies show that some types of cancer cells metabolize fructose to increase their growth.[63] High-fructose corn syrup is manufactured by altering corn's starch molecules which leaves the fructose molecules "free and unbound," so they are easily absorbed by the body. This may be the reason for the steady rise in obesity and diabetes.[64] In the U.S. we consume about 55 pounds of high-fructose corn syrup per person per year.[65]

Do cancer cells need sugar to survive? Yes! Cancer cells have an insatiable appetite for sweets. A person with high levels of blood sugar is actually feeding the cancer cells. Studies on the cancer risk in Korean men and women have shown that the higher the fasting serum glucose level, the higher the incidence of cancer.[66] This was also observed among experimental animals fed a high-sugar diet had twice the tumor incidence as the control group.[67]

What about synthetic sweeteners? Let's look at aspartame, a common artificial sweetener. In the late 1970, animal studies on synthetic sweeteners showed that they aided the development of brain tumors. Other studies show a dose-dependent incidence of brain tumors – the higher the dose of aspartame, the more brain tumors.[68]

In spite of the adverse results from animal studies, the FDA has approved aspartame for human consumption. Since then, brain lesions, tumors, lymphoma, and other diseases have been linked to the use of synthetic sweeteners.[69] Among the elderly, at least twofold increases in brain cancer incidence were observed over the last two decades.[70] During this same time period, brain tumors in all age groups jumped by greater than ten percent.[71,72]

At the Cesare Maltoni Cancer Research Center in Italy, researchers labeled aspartame as a "multi-potential carcinogenic agent." Their animal study linked aspartame to increased incidence of tumors, lymphomas, leukemia, and transitional cell carcinomas of the renal pelvis and ureter. The researchers called for an urgent reevaluation on the use of aspartame.[73]

Artificial sweeteners are addictive, creating a craving for sweeter and higher fatty foods.[74] Many processed products contain artificial sweeteners. Aspartame is found in several commercial sweeteners as NutraSweet, Equal, and Spoonful. Other synthetic sweeteners include sucralose (Splenda); and acesulfame-k (Sunette, Sweet & Safe, and

Sweet One). Beware of these sweet-sounding names that can lead to sour consequences!

Let us close cancer's "second mouth," which is refined sugars and synthetic sweeteners, by closing our own mouth to them. Instead refined sugars and synthetic sweeteners, replace them with natural sweeteners (Chapter 15). Be especially vigilant about processed foods, usually in packages, boxes, bottles, cans, or wrapped or unwrapped, with or without labels, because most likely they contain refined sugars, artificial sweeteners, and chemicals.

Refined/Processed Foods: Grains, Legumes, Fats and Oils – Cancer's Third Mouth

A third type of cancer-promoting foods is the refined/processed foods. This includes all food items that have been altered from their original form as grown. It is tragic that most Americans consume more than half of their total calories and nearly 90 percent of their food budget on refined processed foods.

The primary function of food is for nourishment. From a nutritional point of view, the emergence of refined/processed foods has contributed to the degeneration of our own health and our children's health. As the nutritional quality declines, the health consequences concomitantly appear earlier. One in three elementary children is now overweight, one in three girls and one in two boys will get cancer in their life time. For all cancers combined, it appears that boys have a significantly higher rate than girls. Children ages 0-14 years have a significantly lower rate than adolescents, ages 15-19 years. Among the different races, white children have the highest cancer incidence rate.[75] Problems of this magnitude can be dramatically diminished if not largely eliminated.

I believe the reason we are experiencing so many health problems is that we are not eating real foods as grown. Instead of eating plants, we eat that which has been made in plants – manufactured foods with genetically altered ingredients, artificial colors, dyes, flavors, chemical preservatives, flavor enhancers, and synthetic additives.

The food industry knows how to tickle our taste buds, enticing us to exponentially greater consumption of junk foods and beverages. Salty and sweet foods can trigger a "pleasure molecule" in the brain causing some people to eat more. We can get hooked on these super-flavored foods similarly to addiction to opiates and other drugs.[76] How sad that many have become unwitting victims of processed, hyper-flavored fake foods! These nutrient-poor foods are hyper-flavored with enormous amounts of fats, sugars, salt, and spices. With the consumption of nutrient-deficient and toxic-laden foods, we have inadvertently changed our internal environment, negatively impacted our digestion, absorption, and weakened our immune system.

How do refined grains and legumes lead to disease? When whole grains are milled, the outer bran, the endosperm, and the inner germ are stripped of more than 24 known minerals, vitamins, fiber, and other essential nutrients. Even with the restoration of the B-vitamins and iron, valuable proteins and other nutrients cannot be replaced. This results in a product with less than 20 percent of its nutritional value in the original whole grain kernel.

Moreover, toxic chemicals are added during milling: chlorine to control mold, potassium bromate as dough conditioners, and benzoyl peroxide bleach to whiten the flour. Thus we consume these nutritionally deficient refined products loaded with chemicals that are addictive and wreak havoc on our health. We are overstuffed, yet undernourished. How ironic that we pay additional money at the health food stores to buy back the bran and wheat germ that refining had removed! There is no way that we can replicate what is in the unprocessed whole foods with processed supplements!

Refined foods include white flour and products made from white wheat flour, such as pasta, noodles, breads, pies, cakes, muffins, cookies, pizzas, and white rice, plus many similar items made from processed grains. Likewise, beans and legumes that have been processed into flour and powder are also considered nutritionally inferior. On the other hand, whole unprocessed foods are not only nourishing, but a daily necessity.

Do processed foods and beverages cause blood sugar surge? Yes, processed foods and beverages can cause a spike in the blood glucose level in the same way as refined sugar. In addition, most refined products contain artificial colors which may be carcinogenic. A recent article reported that caramel coloring of colas is carcinogenic.[77] In the U.S. the average person drinks 412 (8-ounce) cokes per year. Are we so addicted to willingly gulp down nearly 40,000 extra calories containing possible carcinogens? Drinking that amount of cokes translates into a weight gain of 11 pounds in a year, 22 pounds in two years, 55 pounds in five years....

How do refined foods feed cancer? Refined foods feed cancer because they lack nutrients and fiber. Most commercially prepared products contribute only empty calories and chemical additives. Frequent consumption of such items will compromise our immune system by creating an ideal environment for cancer development.

Loss of nutrients: Eating refined foods has the same effect as eating refined sugar. Since fiber and vital nutrients have been removed, refined foods can spike the blood sugar levels quickly and cause a surge of insulin and insulin-like growth factor that stimulate abnormal cell growth.[60]

Loss of fiber: Studies have shown that people consuming high-fiber foods had lower rates of colorectal and breast cancer.[9] We know that fiber has the ability to bind with toxic chemicals, cholesterol, sex hormones, waste products, and xenoestrogens (man-made hormone disruptors) and thereby eliminating them from the body.[78] In addition, fiber slows down glucose absorption to avoid the glucose surges that feed cancer.

One needs to be vigilant in avoiding refined/processed food and beverages, such as white pasta, white rice, white breads, rolls, sugary-fatty pastries, and other commercial baked products; candy-coated-breakfast cereals; and high-fructose corn syrup products often found in commercial ketchup, dressings, sauces, gravies, frozen food, and beverages; and canned, bottled, boxed, and wrapped snacks, beverages, and other highly processed convenience items.

Today, our Western diet comprised mainly animal foods and refined foods. Only 7 percent of our present diet comes from whole plant foods.[79] On the other hand, the unprocessed plant-based foods provide a *complete package of nutrients* that gives life and delivers energy. Nothing is added. Nothing is missing.

Refined Fats and Oils

Fats are essential components of our cells and tissues. The best dietary fats are those found naturally in whole foods such as avocados, olives, coconuts, raw nuts, and seeds. However, when fats are refined they can produce serious health consequences.

Most fats and oils are extracted with chemical solvents, at high temperatures, bleached, and deodorized. Refined fats and oils create damaging free radicals that can wreak havoc in our body particularly in cancer. Furthermore, refined fats and oils contain zero fiber, devoid of nutrients, and full of empty calories. Refined fats and oils are found in nearly all processed products.

Overheated fats are hard to digest. Why? Fats need to be emulsified in order to be properly digested and assimilated by the body. If fats have been heated in excess of 125°F, the pancreatic digestive juices cannot adequately act upon or metabolize the food. Instead, these foods can clog the blood vessels, create inflammation, generate destructive free radicals, and produce toxic wastes.[80]

Refined fats and oils are associated with cancer. How?

They suppress the immune system and increase metastasis: Vegetable oils and fish oil suppress the immune system, and increase tumor metastasis. These oils actually promote the spread of some cancers.[81,82]

Heated fats and oils produce carcinogenic compounds and are pro-inflammatory: When oil reaches the temperature at which it begins to smoke, it becomes damaged. Damaged molecules then create free radicals in the body that are potentially carcinogenic.[83]

Fats transport carcinogens in the blood stream: The more fatty foods we eat, the more fat will be in the blood. Fats carry carcinogens to the organs.[84] Carcinogens tend to store in the body's fatty tissues.

Fats increase cancer risks in women and men: Fat is known to affect sex hormones in both men and women and also to increase the risk of breast, uterus, and cervical cancer in women, and prostate cancer in men. Research show that the less fat consumption, the less risk for cancer. Higher fat consumption increases risk for cancer.[12]

The use of vegetable oils has been implicated in skin cancer. A study conducted by the Arizona Cancer Center reported that increased levels of arachidonic acid were associated with increased skin squamous cell carcinoma among 656 participants.[85] Arachidonic acid occurs in animal fats; but it can also be formed from vegetable oils.[86]

Fats and oils contribute to fat calories: Approximately 40 percent of our calories come from fatty foods such as meats, poultry, fish, seafood, milk, dairy products, salad dressings, gravies, fried foods, and other commercially prepared products, including cookies, crackers, chips, breakfast bars and innumerable other items containing refined fats and oils. Dietary fat includes all types from both animal and vegetable sources.

Fats and oils are cholesterol in disguise: Vegetable oils also contain saturated fat, which is dubbed as "cholesterol in disguise."[87] Dean Ornish, MD, explains that vegetable oils will "stimulate your liver to make more cholesterol than your body needs and ends up clogging arteries." Hydrogenated vegetable oils (trans-fats) are "particularly efficient at clogging arteries and depriving your body of oxygen."[87]

Sometimes we may be deceiving ourselves when we eat a big salad with two tablespoons of salad dressing – thinking we included a healthy salad today. We may even forgo a slice pizza, French fries, one cup ice cream or even a piece of apple pie. But all of these items contain the same fat equivalent as two tablespoons of vegetable oil salad dressing! So beware! But wait... this is not to say that pizza, fries, ice cream or pies are necessarily any better!

Form a habit of *reading labels* on all commercially prepared products. Ingredients are listed in descending order by quantity or by weight. Usually you will find white flour, sugar, fats and oils in the beginning of the list. There are also chemical additives listed at the end. If the label lists more than five ingredients or if a fifth grader cannot pronounce the ingredients, put the item back on the shelf.

Bottom Line -- Certain Foods Contribute To Cancer Risks

The cancer promoters include animal foods, refined sugars and synthetic sweeteners, refined/processed grains and legumes, and refined fats and oils. Those who consume cancer promoters have more carcinogens, synthetic hormones, and toxic chemicals in their body. Remember cancer's three mouths. Do not feed them!

Conditions Cancer Cells Love

To conclude this chapter, let me summarize conditions in which cancer cells thrive:[88]

High Acidity: Cancer cells prefer an acidic environment, which come from consuming animal foods. The average person in this country consumes a highly acidic diet. Plant-based foods, on the other hand, provide more alkaline conditions in the body. Alkaline foods furnish valuable minerals and nutrients, increase energy production, and enhance the body's repair and renewal of diseased cells. In addition, alkaline foods can detoxify heavy metals and deter tumor survival. Plant foods are protective against cancers.

Poor circulation, low nutrient and oxygen levels: Cancer cells can thrive without oxygen. In fact, they prefer an anaerobic (oxygen-free) condition.[89] An oxygen deficient environment can cause normal cells to mutate and become cancerous. When blood vessels become clogged from animal foods an ideal condition for the nutrient-starved and oxygen-deprived cells to mutate and turn cancerous.

High blood sugar from refined sugars and starch: Cancer cells are sugar guzzlers, consuming 18 times more sugar than normal cells because they have more glucose receptors on their cell surface than healthy cells. However, if we keep the blood glucose at normal levels, then cancer growth is slowed down.

High cholesterol level from animal-based foods: A positive correlation exists between total serum cholesterol levels and cancer mortality.[90] When animals were on a cholesterol free diet, there was a significant increase in their survival and a reduction in the incidence of metastases.[91] Studies have also found that cancer cells have higher demands for cholesterol than healthy cells. In other words, *cholesterol fuels cancer.*[92] Cancer cells have an unquenchable appetite for fatty foods and love not only sugary foods but fatty foods as well. Both animal fats and vegetable fats are risk factors in many types of cancers.[93]

High sex hormones from eating animal foods and refined fats and oils: High fatty foods and body fat are the main contributors in high levels of sex hormones. The higher these hormones, the greater the chance of getting cancers of the breast, prostate, and other hormone related cancers. With today's factory farming practices, drinking milk and eating dairy products may heighten the risk of some cancers.[94,95] Milk from cows late in pregnancy contains 33 times more estrogen and 10 times more progesterone than milk from non-pregnant cows.

We Can Stop Cancer

What we eat influences our risks and our chances for recovery from cancer. Our cancer-prone body comes as a direct result of eating a diet high in animal protein, cholesterol, fat, sugar, genetically altered hormones, refined/processed foods, acidic levels, and low in nutrient oxygen levels. But we can stop cancer, simply by our food choices. We can reduce our risk by changing our body's cancer-prone condition to an "anti-cancer" environment. Those who consume cancer promoter foods have more carcinogens, synthetic hormones, and toxic chemicals in their bodies. Remember cancer's three mouths 癌. You can stop cancer by closing your mouth to:

• Animal foods

- Sugary foods
- Refined/processed foods

In later chapters, I will discuss in detail our three-step nutritionally sound program, the 3 "R" Diet. It is a nutrition-based program that can reduce cancer risks and reverse cancer. But first, allow me to tell you my nutrition research with chlorella, a green algae grown on recycled water.

CHAPTER 11

MY NUTRITION RESEARCH

My (Esther's) dilemma upon entering college in Michigan was what field to pursue. I finally decided to major in nutrition. To me the word "nutrition" was synonymous with the word "protein." And protein was synonymous with good health. The critical factor of protein was underscored over and over again by our professors. They often reminded us that adequate dietary protein automatically ensures a well-balanced diet. A balanced diet then equates adequate protein intake, so I thought.

In one of the classes, I was assigned to give a nutrition talk on the importance of protein to third graders in a local elementary school. On that day, I made a dramatic entrance, dressed in an old oversized outfit from a thrift shop into the class room as "Old Mother Hubbard" amidst a ripple of giggles. Donned with a loosely fitting hat that unexpectedly dropped to my nose and knocked off my glasses, I blindly bumped into a file cabinet with a loud bang. A spontaneous outburst of laughter erupted! (Believe me, it was an accident). Dragging out the syllables, I swaggered and uttered the familiar nursery rhyme –

"Old Mother Hubbard
Went to the cupboard
To get her poor doggie a bone,
When she got there
The cupboard was bare
So the poor little doggie had none.

Then I trotted toward the old upright piano and started playing a familiar tune "Oh, My Darling Clementine." Using my made-up lyrics for this occasion, I taught the students to sing: "Let's eat protein, let's eat protein, let's eat protein every day. It will make you strong and healthy, let's eat protein every day." After singing, I shed my hideous attire and turned on the electric skillet. With eager anticipation, these third graders watched as I demonstrated how to make a high protein veggie-burger. I used dehydrated soy and wheat gluten bits combined with eggs and milk powder for additional protein, then pan-fried the burgers in hot sizzling oil. My classmates helped to assemble them on buttered white buns, topped with generous globs of mayonnaise and other condiments. The third graders loved the veggie-burgers by their ketchup-mayonnaise-smeared smiles and finger-licking applause!

Reality set in when I began a 12-month dietetic internship after completing my B.A. degree. I was assigned to the cancer wards at the Los Angeles County Medical Center, one of the largest medical centers at that time. One can easily get lost in that colossal building with a jungle-like maze of long, dimly-lit corridors. Each day I timidly visited patients and evaluated their dietary needs. After carefully planning balanced meals with high protein in-between feedings for the cancer patients, I was shocked to see their food trays came back untouched. I felt helpless as I saw them suffering from severe nausea, vomiting, and retching with pain days on end. Soon cancer had taken their lives. Had medicine failed them? Did I fail them nutritionally? I pondered.

Shortly after my enrollment in graduate school at the University of California in Berkeley, my nutrition professor's sister died of cancer, a young mother with 3 children. A few months later my professor's husband died of a massive heart attack. Was their diet balanced? Surely they consumed adequate protein. I was baffled.

The protein quality of green algae

For my master's degree research project I chose one topic that particularly piqued my curiosity – "The protein quality of waste-grown green algae." I was intrigued – how can seaweed contain protein? And of all places, algae grown on recycled waste-water?

I delved into my research – comparing the protein quality of this type of algae (chlorella) with casein (milk protein), the gold standard of measuring the biologic value of a food substance. For my research, the waste-grown green algae powder was supplied by the University of California Sanitary Engineering Research Laboratory. I prepared the experimental rat chow combining the algae with oats, wheat, and peanuts. These combinations were fed to several groups of animals; then we measured their growth with the growth of the control animals on the milk casein diet. Results showed that the waste-grown green algae when combined with whole grains and peanuts did support growth of the experimental animals. Our study was published in the *Journal of Nutrition.*[1]

I also made cookies using the green algae powder taste-tested by over 100 undergraduate nutrition students. Their evaluation comments varied: "a bid sea-weedy taste," to "O.K.," to "yummy!" especially those made in combination with peanut butter. Buoyed by the results from my animal research and the positive feedback from the taste-testing panel, I took a big bag of the green algae powder home to my newly-wed husband. He surprised me one evening by cooking a whole meal using the algae powder! Even today we are still taking a green powder in smoothies for breakfast every so often.

For the first time, I realized that plant proteins can support growth. It was not until many years later, that I began to recognize the nutritional superiority in plant-based foods.

Being young and naïve, yet to have chosen to study the protein quality of green algae, might have elevated me a bit ahead of my time! Of course, back then, I didn't know that chlorella, unicellular green algae contain high levels of chlorophyll, protein, including all nine essential amino acids, enzymes, vitamins, and trace minerals. I also did not know that chlorella is rich in phytochemicals useful against cancer. Furthermore, I was ignorant of the effect of milk protein on the risk for cancer.

However, now many years later, the outstanding research by Dr. T. Colin Campbell provides convincing data that *all animal protein, including the milk protein (casein) promotes cancer.* He stated that "Casein, and very likely all animal proteins, may be the most relevant cancer-causing substances that we consume."[2]

Nutrition science has also shifted considerably from my college days learning that a high protein diet equates a healthy diet to now recognizing that protein intake can indeed be adequately supplied by a plant-based diet.

Sometime later, I read a statement from an old dilapidated book that helped to sharpen my focus on using food as medicine, and yes, perhaps even in stopping cancer. In 1314 A.D., an imperial physician in China, Hu Se-Hui stated: "Food alone cures many diseases."[3] Oh, food alone cures many diseases? Is that possible? After reading such an unexpected statement, I began an earnest search for the healing powers in foods. That search opened my eyes for a paradigm shift in preventing and reversing cancer.

CHAPTER 12

PHYTOTHERAPY – CRUX OF THE MATTER

Phytotherapy is food therapy. We use the unprocessed plant-based whole foods for treating diseases. In fact, a plant-based diet may be the "breakthrough" for stopping cancer. Such a diet provides nutrients to starving cells, tissues and organs, while simultaneously boost a healthy immune system to stave off cancer.

How so? It is through the multiple "phyto-actions" of phytochemicals in plant-based whole foods. These "phyto-actions" are the very essence of healing! The phytochemicals have the innate ability to bring about a concomitant death of cancer cells while simultaneously fortifying our normal cells with powerful "phyto-ammunitions" to destroy and wipe out cancer. No other therapy can initiate such a dual effect! Thus, based on the enormous potential power in phytochemicals, we can explain and establish that phytotherapy is effective in stopping cancer.

Even though cancer is a complex disease, yet scientists have discovered that substances in food can either *promote* or *interfere* with the disease process. In earlier chapters, we mentioned certain foods (animal foods, refined sugar, refined grains/legumes, and refined fats and oils) promote cancer development. In this chapter our focus is on the "cancer fighters." We will first discuss the phytochemicals' capability as cancer fighters. Then, we will also address the question – why and how phytotherapy can stop cancer.

What are phytochemicals?

The word "phyto" is derived from the Greek word for plants. Phytochemicals refer to the chemicals that are found in whole plant foods (fruits, vegetables, grains, beans, legumes, seeds, and herbs). It is well-known that a plant produces chemicals to protect itself from the environment, but research has demonstrated that these plant chemicals can also protect humans against diseases.

How do the phytochemicals work?

Phytochemicals protect our body against damages through the following actions:

1. Acting as antioxidants to keep free radicals from damaging our cells; and reduce the risk of certain cancers.
2. Producing hormonal actions that imitate human estrogens (phytoestrogens) and help to reduce diseases.
3. Stimulating enzymes that can suppress and inhibit certain undesirable activities and reduce the risk for certain cancers.
4. Interfering with DNA replications; prevent the multiplication of cancer cells.
5. Creating an anti-microbial effect that protect against diseases.[1]

The phytochemicals' multiple actions are precisely why phytotherapy is so effective against cancer.

Do plants have immune system? No, but they use phytochemicals as their defense system. If plants can protect themselves with their phytochemicals, how do they help us in stopping cancer? In chapters 1 and 5, we presented two amazing mechanisms of the phytochemicals' ability to help us through the following ways:

1. Causing the cancer cells (enemies) to commit suicide or programmed death (apoptosis).
2. Feeding nutrients to our immune cells to enhance their potency and function by removing their blindfolds so they can do their job.

Can phytochemicals harm our normal healthy cells? No, phytochemicals do not harm the normal cells because they have *selective* toxicity! It is truly astounding that plant chemicals can destroy only cancer cells and not only spare the normal cells but also nourish them (Chapters 2, 3, & 7)! That's a form of discrimination with precision. Certain phytochemicals will cause cancer cell death (apoptosis), while other phytochemicals serve as nutrients to strengthen our immune cells. In chemotherapy, toxic chemicals indiscriminately kill both cancer and normal cells. Phytotherapy is chemotherapy, without the side effects.

Of course, using food for treating cancer seems foreign to many people. I recall an oncologist friend with colon cancer jokingly declared, "If anyone tells me to eat some greens to cure cancer, he needs his head examined!" Later he died of cancer.

Some years ago, I chuckled at this caption in a magazine: "Take one head of broccoli and call me in the morning." Today broccoli no longer is the butt of jokes.

In fact, health professionals, scientists, and researchers have begun to recognize the power of food in preventing and healing diseases including cancer. Compelling evidence from a wide range of studies by multiple disciplines indicate that a plant-based diet can dramatically cut the risk of all types of cancer. According to Joel Fuhrman, MD, a person can reduce the odds of getting cancer "by 60 to 80 percent through diet alone."[2]

This same sentiment was also expressed by Dr. Richard Beliveau, who stated, "All the studies on cancer and nutrition point to eating plant-based foods for their phytonutrients and other special compounds."[3]

How do whole plant-based foods help to stop cancer?

- Plant-based whole foods contain thousands of healing phytochemicals
- Plant-based whole foods are naturally low in fat
- Plant-based whole foods are mostly alkaline
- Plant-based whole foods detoxify

Plant-based whole foods contain thousands of healing phytochemicals: Establishing the exact number of healing plant chemicals in whole foods is difficult because of the enormous number of phytochemicals and the complexity of their activities. Since sophisticated measuring devices have been developed, more phytonutrients are being identified. Still thousands of unknown, unnamed and, yes, undiscovered ones have yet to emerge.

What we do know is that the whole unprocessed foods provide synergistic benefits exponentially better than the processed synthetic isolated supplements. Our job is simply to eat the unprocessed whole foods that support the body's own healing.

Thousands of phytochemicals are present in virtually all fresh fruits, vegetables, whole legumes, whole grains, nuts, and seeds. For example, a carrot contains hundreds phytochemicals. We have much evidence from observations of cultures in which the diet consists mainly from plant sources with lower rates of cancers and heart diseases. The American Cancer Society's 2012 nutrition guidelines recommend a balanced diet with foods from a variety of plant sources along with physical activity and smoking cessation.[4,5] Diets rich in fruits, vegetables, legumes, and grains not only reduce the risks of cancer, but also increase survival.

Phytochemicals in whole plant-based foods are non-toxic medicines providing the following healing activities by:

- Blocking the carcinogens before they do any damage
- Supplying protective enzymes
- Neutralizing destructive molecules
- Dismantling the undesirable hormones by blocking the receptor sites
- Furnishing nutrients and other substances in fighting cancer

In other words, thousands of naturally occurring substances in whole plant foods feed and fortify our body's immune cells as well as nourish all cells to combat cancer. For example, researchers have shown that greater intake of vegetables and fruits were associated with a decreased risk of breast cancer. That is, the more vegetables and fruits consumed the less is the risk for breast cancer. Dark green leafy vegetables, cruciferous vegetables, carrots, tomatoes, banana, watermelon, papaya, cantaloupe were shown to significantly lower the risk of breast cancer.[6]

Plant-based whole foods are naturally low in fat: Whole grains, whole beans, fruits, and vegetables are naturally low in fat. These whole foods provide essential nutrients as protein, complex carbohydrates, natural fats, vitamins, minerals, fiber, antioxidants, and phytochemicals. The unprocessed grains, beans, fruits, and vegetables add texture, flavor, and satiety value to our meals without the use of refined fats and oils.

Most plant-based whole foods are low in fat with a few exceptions, such as avocados, olives, coconuts, nuts, and seeds. These higher fat foods can be judiciously included in the diet, but they are best in the raw form (raw nuts and raw seeds). For its many functions, the body needs naturally occurring fats which are adequately supplied by whole plant foods. But refined/processed fats and oils should be avoided.

As mentioned earlier, all refined/processed foods should be avoided including items made from white flour, other refined grains, and processed beans, and legumes. Most commercially prepared products contain considerable amounts of refined sugar and fat.

Plant-based whole foods are mostly alkaline: What we eat affects the acidity or alkalinity of the blood which is measured by the pH scale. The normal pH of blood is slightly alkaline, about 7.35 - 7.45. Our blood pH must stay within this narrow range for optimum health and for our cells to function properly. Most plant foods are alkaline. When the body's pH level is balanced with an abundant supply of alkaline minerals from fruits and vegetables, then the body is able to repair damaged cells, increase energy production, and detoxify, all necessary in stopping cancer. Fortunately, we have multiple buffer systems that keep our pH within the normal range, but eating improper foods can cause a deficiency in our reserves.

Acid forming foods create health problems. A diet high in acid forming foods (animal protein, sugar, refined and processed foods, alcohol, caffeine, and sodas) can shift the pH toward more acidic range. Our Western diet tends to be acidic. Most diets around the world also shift as people consume more animal and processed foods. A diet high in acid-forming foods can lead to a higher risk of osteoporosis, fractures, kidney stones plus other negative health consequences. Unless the body's pH level is slightly alkaline, it is difficult for the body to heal from many chronic diseases, particularly cancer.

Cancer cells prefer acidic environment. Cancer cells thrive in an acidic environment. All animal foods, refined processed foods, and sugary beverages are acidic. But we can change to a more alkaline environment so cancer cells cannot survive. The best way to achieve balance is to eat more alkaline foods than acid foods. This means that we need to eat approximately 80 percent alkaline-forming foods (most fruits and vegetables); and about 20 percent acid-forming foods (most whole grains and beans). By continuously supplying alkaline elements in our diet, we can turn sick cells back to normal healthy cells.

Plant-based whole foods detoxify: Plant-based whole foods are potent detoxifiers. Most of the unprocessed plant foods contain fiber and alkaline minerals that are capable of neutralizing and eliminating toxic wastes from the body. Dietary fiber is highly protective for colon cancer.[7] Additionally, fiber can help normalize blood sugar and reduce blood cholesterol, both of which feed cancer. Remember, cancer cells love sweets and fatty foods. Whole plant foods also contain high water content which can help to dissolve toxins and flush out inorganic deposits. Animal foods, on the other hand, contain zero fiber that can lead to constipation, and increase toxicity in the body.

How do we incorporate phytotherapy?

For a person with cancer, regardless of the treatment choices (chemotherapy, radiation, surgery, or any other therapies), *dietary change is critical.* Without switching from "cancer-promoters" to foods that are "cancer-fighters," it remains doubtful whether one can achieve a permanent cancer cure.

Phytotherapy involves two steps:

1. **NO RATS** – we need to stop eating cancer-promoters which I call **RATS** – a simple acronym to help us remember which foods we need to avoid:

   R = **R**efined foods
   A = **A**nimal foods
   T = **T**oxins (artificial sweeteners, additives, and GMOs)
   S = **S**ugar

Cancer promoting foods include all highly **refined** processed fats, oils, grains, beans, legumes; all **animal**-based foods (meat, poultry, fish, sea foods, eggs, cow's milk, and dairy products); all **toxins** such as artificial sweeteners, chemical additives such as MSG, other flavor enhancers, synthetic colors, dyes, preservatives, thickeners, fillers, and genetically modified organisms; and refined **sugars** (corn syrup, high fructose corn syrup, and more). Most commercially prepared foods are loaded with **RATS**!

2. **BGFVR** – we need to eat cancer-fighter foods. Just remember to do yourself a **BIG FAVOR** (remove the vowels for BGFVR):

   BGFV = R

   > **B**eans and legumes
   > **G**rains
   > **F**ruits
   > **V**egetables
   > **R**ight diet

Every day eat the cancer fighters found in beans, grains, fruits, and vegetables for the **Right** diet (Chapter 15). Only plant-based whole foods are cancer fighters, as they deliver thousands of healing nutrients to our cells. This is *nutrition-based medicine* – strikingly powerful, yet without adverse side effects. Regardless of what other therapies one may choose, a plant-based diet is the single, most powerful strategy in preventing and reversing cancer. In the next chapter, we will discuss the three "R" diet to stop cancer.

CHAPTER 13

THE REVERSE DIET

In this chapter, I will provide some general guidelines for our three-step nutritional program – the 3 "R" Diets:

1. The Reverse Diet
2. The Recovery Diet
3. The Right Diet

The nutritional program consists of a graduated three step-process, beginning with the Reverse Diet for those who are at a serious stage of the illness, whose health is in jeopardy. The focus is to remove toxins out of the body, and replenish it with healing nutrients. This is a short term, first step to stopping cancer, with a time frame varying from a few days to a week or longer, depending on the patient.

The second stage, the Recovery Diet, continues the healing process but with less dietary limitation, and the third stage is the Right Diet which is sustainable for optimal health.

We encourage the use of fresh raw fruits and raw vegetables, whole grains, whole legumes, whole beans, and unprocessed unrefined plant foods. If feasible, use organic produce and organic products, particularly for those containing high levels of contaminants (Chapter 16). Within these guidelines, this program is flexible and may be adapted to fit individual needs, preferences, and schedules.

Let us begin with Step 1 – The Reverse Diet.

How can toxins be removed and nutrients replenished?

The best way to remove cellular toxins and to replenish nutrients is to drink freshly extracted fruit and vegetable juices. Juice therapy is the most efficient method to remove toxins and to replenish starving cells with vital nutrients.

During the initial period, our digestive system cannot handle so much bulk, let alone assimilate all the necessary healing nutrients that raw vegetables and fruit contain. Only about 35 percent of the nutrients ingested are assimilated by most people, but that percentage spirals down to only about one percent by those who are sick. However, in the form of raw juices, one can assimilate up to 92 percent of these essential nutrients. A pioneer in juice therapy, H. E. Kirschner, MD, stated: "The juices of the plant, like the blood of the body contain all the elements that build and nourish."[1]

Raw juice therapy is the quickest way to reverse a diseased condition. At the same time, we also need to reduce the work load of the digestive system. Digestion is one of the most energy demanding processes. By drinking juices, we allow the digestive organs to conserve its energy for maximum healing.

The Reverse Diet Menu - a typical day's fresh juice diet

The juices can be taken at intervals of one to two hours as suggested:

- Upon arising – water or miso broth or herb tea (red clover) with small amount of freshly squeezed lemon juice
- 1-2 hours later – Fresh fruit juice with green powder or green liquid supplement (any organically grown whole plant food and herb concentrate in powder or liquid form)
- 1-2 hours later – Fresh vegetable juice
- 1-2 hours later – Fresh vegetable juice
- 1-2 hours later – Water or miso broth or herb tea with lemon
- 1-2 hours later – Fresh vegetable juice

- 1-2 hours later – Fresh vegetable juice with green powder or liquid supplement
- 1-2 hours later – Fresh vegetable juice
- 1-2 hours later – Water or miso broth or herb tea with lemon
- 1-2 hours later – Fresh vegetables or fresh fruit juice

In addition, it is recommended that a person take a natural herbal cleanse or do an enema to keep bowels open.

How does the body eliminate toxins?

Cancer is linked to toxicity – toxic food, toxic air/water/environment, and toxic habits; fortunately, our bodies are equipped with five organs that eliminate toxins. We coined the word – "KILLS" to depict these five organs: kidneys, intestines, lungs, liver, and skin. If these organs are compromised, then the built-up toxicities can kill us. Often during serious illnesses, our elimination organs are not up to par. Sometimes because of a lifetime of neglected habits, one can develop chronic diseases as a result of toxic accumulation. In this section we will discuss one of the most important organs of elimination, the large intestines – the colon.

A constipated colon can cause all kinds of problems, the cause of which are often difficult to identify. These include allergies, bad breath, headaches, gastritis, heart burn, polyps, colitis, liver diseases, and cancer. The first step towards recovery is to keep the colon clean. When the colon is healthy, approximately 60 to 80 percent of health problems generally disappear. Here are tips for a healthy colon:

1. Take time every day to empty the body's waste.
2. Drink more water.
3. Exercise to improve muscular contractions.
4. Manage stress. When stressed, anxious or worried, all bodily organs, especially the colon, are affected.
5. When necessary, use natural herbal cleansing or an enema to keep bowels emptied.

Which juicer should I buy?

There are many fruit and vegetable juicers on the market. Choose one that best fit your needs and budget. Current prices range from $70 to over $500. The juicer must be able to separate the pulp (fiber) from the juice as the juices are being extracted. Follow the manufacturer's instructions on the proper operation and care of the juicer.

How do I make fresh fruit and vegetable juices?

Choose organic produce, if available. Organic produce is grown without chemical additives and toxic pesticides. Always store the produce in the refrigerator. When ready to make the juice do the following:

1. Scrub the fruits and vegetables clean.
2. Discard the outer leaves of non-organic produce; peel any waxed fruit or vegetables.
3. Cut produce to small pieces to fit into the feeder chute.
4. Leafy greens, sprouts, wheat grass can be rolled up into small balls, and push through the feeder with carrots or other firm vegetables.
5. Soft fruits can be pushed through with firm apples or carrots.

What kind of juices should I use? Any fresh fruit or fresh vegetables in season can be used for juices. If a person is sensitive to sweet fruits, one can dilute it with water or use just vegetable juices.

Due to the strong flavors in the green vegetables (spinach, collards, mustard greens, wheat grass, barley greens, kale, broccoli, cabbage, and others), the proportions should be one-fourth (¼) cup of these greens to a pint (2 cups) of carrot juice. For every 5 pounds of organic carrots, it will yield approximately 5-6 cups of juice. Other vegetables such as beets, bell peppers, cucumbers, celery, zucchini, yellow squash, and lettuce can also be included. Carrots should be used as a base for other vegetables. Pungent vegetables, such as onions, garlic, ginger, and hot peppers can be added. They should be in *miniscule* quantities and as tolerated by the individual.

Wheatgrass juice can be taken in small quantities two or three time a day. Wheatgrass tops any greens in nutrition and in healing. Some prefer to take it with a little lemon juice, while others like to sweeten it with freshly extracted apple juice.

Remember to drink the juices on an empty stomach for quick assimilation. Never drink juices at the end of a meal.

How much juice should I drink? One must remember that during the acute stage, a person may be too sick to consume large quantities of juices. It is advisable to start with small quantities, beginning with a spoonful, gradually increasing as tolerated.

Initially one should aim for one pint (2 cups) daily, and then work up from "two to eight pints or more," according to Dr. Norman Walker, one of the most authoritative scientists on nutrition and health.[2] Drinking more juices bring quicker results, but one must be patient – healing takes time. Starting out sickly as a child, Dr. Walker was one of the first to discover the health benefits in freshly squeezed juices. It was reported that he wrote his last book at the age of 115; and lived an active life to 119 years of age!

Why drink miso broth? Miso is an enzyme-rich fermented soybean paste that provides many health benefits. Miso contains isoflavones which are believed to fight cancer cells, and decrease risk of breast cancer, prostate, lung, and colon cancer.[3] Studies in Japan show that consuming just one bowl of miso soup a day cuts the risk of breast cancer. It also provides beneficial bacteria and valuable enzymes necessary for good digestion particularly during the acute stage of an illness.[4]

What can be done for nausea? Sipping organic apple cider vinegar or chewing on fresh ginger slices often relieves nausea. Ginger also reduces inflammation. In addition, studies with ovarian cancer cells show that ginger causes the *in vitro* cancer cells to die by either committing suicide (apoptosis) or by attacking themselves (autophagy).[5]

What can I expect while on the Reverse Diet?

During this period, the body may experience unexpected symptoms that one may not expect. A person may experience more pain, digestive and respiratory discomforts, and just a general "not good feeling." Do not think that the juices are making you ill. Remember, the aim is to quickly remove toxins out and put nutrients in. Freshly squeezed juices are both cleansing and healing. The discomforts one may experience are an indication that the body is responding to the regenerative powers in the juices. This condition is described as the "healing crisis." Cutting back on the amount of juice may minimize the discomforts. In time the body will adjust to the cleansing and such discomforts dissipates.

Why remove pulp? Why not eat the whole fruit and vegetables? As mentioned earlier, digestion is one of the most energy demanding activities. At this critical period, a diet of solid foods places an enormous burden on our digestive system, but a juice diet minimizes the work load of our digestive organs while simultaneously delivering the healing nutrients into cells quickly. Thus a fiber-free juice can be digested and assimilated in a matter of minutes with a minimum burden on the digestive system. Fresh juice therapy can be compared with an intravenous feeding. I consider juice therapy as a powerful "nutritional" I.V. minus the needle!

How long should one stay on the fresh juice diet? As soon as a person is able to tolerate solid foods, one can progress to Step 2 – the Recovery Diet. Generally five days to a week or two – should be adequate, but again, one must monitor the individual response to the juices and readiness for solid foods. Some people progress at a much slower pace than others. It is prudent to allow for such differences.

What if my skin color turns yellow? Good! Be assured that it is not the carrot pigment that is coming through the skin. It would be just as ludicrous to see the red beets or green spinach pigments coming through the skin. With one exception, however, the red pigment from red beets can show up in the urine and feces. Do not be alarmed. Since these juices have started an internal house cleaning, any yellow or brown appears on the skin is an indication that the liver is releasing toxins, bile, and other waste products. In time, the discoloration disappears.

One morning as soon as I opened our clinic door, a patient, a first-year medical student, looking anxious blurted out,

"I passed out blood in my stools this morning."

"How do you feel?" I asked.

"Fine, but what's wrong with me?"

Knowing that he did not eat fish or any animal products, I asked, "Did you eat some beets yesterday?" Immediately, his face relaxed, and he joyfully bounced out of the office heading to his 8:00 am anatomy class!

CHAPTER 14

THE RECOVERY DIET

"Health is important for all the world
It's like a diamond or a pearl
It makes you do things you should
Run to make you fit
Don't be lazy, don't just sit
Enjoy the world all over you
Because this poem is healthy and true."

Kyra Kaya, 8 years old

In this chapter we will also focus on some essential lifestyle habits in addition to the Recovery Diet. As part of recovery, indispensable lifestyle choices also need to become part of our daily routine. When lifestyle changes are incorporated, one can recover.

Scientists have discovered that a plant-based diet, exercise, stress management, and meaningful social involvement can prolong life. They measured the lengths of the telomeres of men with prostate cancer. Telomeres are the protective caps on the ends of chromosomes (part of cell nucleus) that affect how quickly cells age. The shorter the telomeres the more quickly the cells die.

Researchers followed 35 men with early-stage prostate cancer for five years. Ten in the group engaged in a plant-based diet, a moderate exercise plan which included walking 30 minutes, 6 days a week, stress reduction with yoga and meditation, and weekly group support. The other 25 men did not make major lifestyle changes. The 10 in the first group experienced a significant increase in telomere length of 10%, while those who made no changes saw a three percent decrease. The more the participants adhered to the healthy plan, the more dramatic their telomere length increased. Research has linked longer telomeres to slower progression of cancer and higher rates of survival.[1] In this section we will introduce a lifestyle concept known around the world as the NEWSTART program.

What is the NEWSTART® program?

The word "NEWSTART" was first coined by a guest at Weimer Health Education Center located in Northern California.[2] This Center has been helping people in the prevention and reversal of diseases through natural methods since the 1970s. The concept, however, dates back to the dawn of earth's history, as recorded in the first book of the Bible – the Genesis account where God provided a blueprint for us to maintain optimum health.

Perhaps the most notable 20th-century American pioneer in demonstrating the benefits of the Newstart lifestyle is John Harvey Kellogg, MD. He along with the then world renowned Battle Creek Sanitarium in Michigan was most influential in promoting the healthy lifestyle. As early as the 1870s, Dr. Kellogg encouraged a low-fat, low-protein diet with an emphasis on whole grains, fiber-rich foods, fruits, vegetables, and nuts. He also recommended exercise, fresh air, and the importance of cleanliness.[3]

The NEWSTART lifestyle revolves around the following eight areas:

N = Nutrition: By consuming only the most wholesome foods with the highest nutritional values, we are helping to build our health to an optimal level. Proper nutrition heals, and, as explained earlier in this book, it is the key that can starve cancer cells and enhance immune cell function. "You are what you eat" may be an oversimplification, but nonetheless, nutrition is of critical import. Yet nutrition alone is not enough. It is imperative to establish a total lifestyle pattern of health.

E = Exercise: Our bodies need motion. Movement and circulation keep us alive. In spite of today's fast paced society, our bodies are slowed to a comfortable crawl. Many simply do not move anymore which can lead to devastating consequences.

Exercise tones the muscles and organs, increases lymphatic activities, boosts the immune system, and helps with the elimination of waste. Remember, cancer thrives in low-oxygen environment, and even healthy cells can mutate to cancerous condition in a low-oxygen environment (Chapter 10). Regular exercise also reduces anxiety, releases tension, and spurs the brain to pump out endorphins, those naturally occurring peptides in the brain that reduces pain and causes us to feel good.

Daily exercise, preferably outdoors, is a necessity and an integral part of healing. Walking and gardening are two simple ways to increase the blood circulation that carries nutrients to every cell.

The role of diet and physical activity in cancer incidence is well documented. It appears that physically active people have better outcomes against cancer recurrence and progression in several common cancers.[4]

W = Water: Many suffer from chronic dehydration, particularly on the cellular level. Even mild dehydration can alter a person's mood, energy level, and ability to think clearly. If a person experiences headache, fatigue, or irritability, drink some water! Most of the beverages we consume, such as coffee, tea, alcohol, soft drinks, and sport drinks actually contribute further to dehydration. It is estimated that 75% of Americans are chronically dehydrated. In some individuals the thirst sensation is so impaired that it is often mistaken for hunger.[5]

A patient who complained of severe headache after surgery was dispensed the prescribed Tylenol #3. While waiting for the prescription to be filled, he decided to drink some water. After gulping down two glasses of water, his headache disappeared, without Tylenol. Among the elderly, I have noted that those who faithfully swallow their daily quota of pills benefitted more from the water that washed down the pills than the pills themselves.

Can drinking water help in preventing cancer? Epidemiological studies have examined the association between fluid intake and different types of cancer. At this point, the findings remain inconclusive due to inadequate assessment.

However, adequate water intake does have preventive effects on cancers of the bladder, colon, and breast.[6] For bladder cancer, decreased fluid intake and, concomitantly, less frequent urination result in greater concentration of carcinogens in the urine and prolonged time of contact with the bladder mucosa. This is also true with colon cancer. Insufficient fluid intake increases the risk of colon cancer because it decreases bowel transit time which in turn increases mucosal contact with carcinogens. Likewise, the risk of breast cancer increases with inadequate fluid consumption.[6]

Adequate hydration hastens healing. We need to drink enough pure water to keep urine clear. The best time to drink water is between meals, half hour before or 2 hours after. Do not drink water with meals as it dilutes the digestive juice and increases digestion time in the stomach.

Water therapy, or hydrotherapy, for treating illnesses dates back to earlier civilizations. We have found it to be effective for pain and infections, particularly for pain and respiratory infections in cancer patients. For additional information, you may consult the book – *Hydrotherapy for Respiratory Infections* by Benjamin Lau, MD, PhD, 2010.[7]

S = Sunlight: The use of sunlight is known as heliotherapy. Consumer health advocate, Mike Adams, calls sunlight the "miracle" therapy.[8] Without sunlight, practically all form of life ceases.

We depend on the sun for synthesis of vitamins, hormones, and minerals necessary for life. Sunlight is the most reliable way to synthesis vitamin D as its rays penetrate our skin. Vitamin D is a potent anti-cancer medicine made in our own skin.

Recent research shows that the sun's healing rays can prevent a variety of cancers, including prostate, breast, cervical, ovarian, colon, and skin cancers. Sunlight also protects against non-Hodgkin's lymphoma and other cancers.[9,10] Cedric F. Garland, MD, cancer prevention specialist at the Moores Cancer Center at the University of California, San Diego, estimates that 250,000 cases of colorectal cancer and 350,000 cases of breast cancer could be prevented worldwide by exposure to sunlight, through diet, and with vitamin D3 supplements.[11]

Just remember to get a sensible amount sunlight exposure daily. Only 10-15 minutes a day of sun exposure to the arms, legs, hands, face is sufficient to meet the body's requirement. Darker skin may require longer exposure. The sun outshines food as the best source of vitamin D. And it is free. Otherwise to get the vitamin D value of 10 minutes exposure to sunlight, you would have to eat over 6 pounds of shiitake mushrooms, 150 egg yolks, 30 servings of fortified cereal or 30 cups of fortified orange juice![12] If sunlight is not available, one may need to take a vitamin D supplement.

T = Temperance: Temperance means a balanced lifestyle in all areas – eating, exercise, work, study, rest, sleep, recreation, social relationships, and doing good works. Even with good habits, one needs to be temperate, and not over-do a good thing.

A = Air: Fresh air is the most important and vital element for the body. It is composed of nitrogen and oxygen. Without these essential elements, the body would disintegrate. Even though we get nitrogen from the food we eat, the nitrogen from the air is our most constant supply. About 78 percent of the air we breathe is composed of nitrogen gas.

Oxygen is equally essential, for without it we cannot live. Avoid shallow breaths that send stress signals to the brain. Try to breathe deeper to assimilate more oxygen. This will improve digestion, enhance mental alertness, reduce stress, and induce sleep.

R = Rest: Rest and sleep are as important as nutrition. The lack of sleep is a significant health concern. Dr. Walker stated (the man who lived to 119 years of age) that ninety per cent of ailments are attributable to insufficient sleep and rest. We know that the body does most repair and rebuild activities during sleep. Sleep recharges, refreshes, as well as restores emotional equilibrium. More importantly, did you know that lack of sleep can alter your genes?

Inadequate sleep alters the activity of hundreds of human genes. Less than six hours of sound sleep alters the activity of up to 700 genes according to the latest study conducted by researchers at the University of Surrey in England. These genes are associated with response to stress and immunity and the control of inflammation. Getting too little sleep for several nights in a row disrupts hundreds of genes that are essential for good health.[13]

Does sleep affect breast cancer risk? A recent research at the Case Western Reserve University in Cleveland showed that postmenopausal women with breast cancer who routinely sleep less than six hours a night may be twice as likely to have more aggressive breast cancers compared with those who sleep longer hours.[14] Getting enough sleep is necessary for maintaining our circadian rhythm which regulates our body's natural DNA repair. When such circadian rhythm is short-changed, repair is disrupted, and diseases set in.

When is the best time to go to sleep? Sleep before midnight is about twice as refreshing as sleep after midnight. The hours before midnight is time when the body does most of its repair work. You can help the body's healing processes by going to sleep early. You can also optimize your "cancer controlling gene" – p53 gene.

What is the p53 gene? P53 is a gene that regulates the cell cycle by controlling normal cell growth. Were it not for the regulatory activities of the p53 gene, imagine what we might look like with our ever growing noses, fingers, and eye lashes! More importantly, the P53 gene is a tumor suppressing gene – its activity stops the formation of tumors. When there is damage to the DNA of a cell, p53 can stop the cell's continued growth and also trigger cell death to prevent cancer growth. And at the same time, p53 can signal the sick cells to repair the damage.[15] But certain foods and lifestyle habits can harm p53 by affecting its production and efficiency.

What factors can harm the p53 gene?

1. Fried foods
2. Animal foods
3. Sugary foods

4.   Lack of sleep
5.   Stress

Because much of our bodily functioning is cyclic, a regular pattern of adequate sleep in a 24-hour cycle and of rest and rejuvenation (Sabbath) in a seven-day cycle will optimize the regulatory activity of p53 genes as well as our overall health.

T = Trust: Our emotions have tremendous impact on the healing process. Negative emotions including fear, anxiety, anger, and depression compromise the body's ability to fight invaders; conversely, hope, optimism, and courage aid recovery.

Studies have shown that our well-being is influenced by our spiritual beliefs. Although difficult to navigate through the maze of such influences; researchers have uncovered a relationship between the brain and beliefs of individuals who incorporate religious activities in their daily living. Andrew Newberg, MD, a neuroscientist at the University of Pennsylvania, found that those who pray, attend religious services, and are involved in church activities exhibit better immune functions and have a greater likelihood of increased health and longevity.[16]

Often when encountering someone burdened with anxiety, discouragement, grief, I would feel helpless. What could I possibly offer? Yet by the end of the conversation, this is what I often heard: "You don't know how much you have helped me. I feel so much better now!" Although I had felt so inadequate, the person felt better. Through the years, I have come to the conclusion that even though no quick-fix solution may be had, just being available to listen, to support, and to encourage means much. Often just conveying that I care and, more importantly, that we have a loving Father in heaven who cares often brings such peace and hope and courage. I would like to share a few Bible texts that have been particularly helpful.

"Fear not; for I am with you;.... I will strengthen you, yes, I will help you, I will uphold you with My righteous right hand." Isaiah 41:10*

"For I know the thoughts that I think toward you....thoughts of peace and not of evil, to give you a future and a hope." Jeremiah 29:11*

".... casting all your care upon Him, for He cares for you." I Peter 5:7*

"My grace is sufficient for you, for My strength is made perfect in weakness." 2 Corinthians 12:9*

"...we shall live with Him by the power of God toward you." 2 Corinthians 13:4*

*Scriptures taken from the New King James Version. Copyright c 1982 by Thomas Nelson, Inc. Used by permission. All rights reserved.

When trust seems to vanish, the Lord God never fails. Our heavenly Father has a personal concern for each one of us. He has a thousand ways to help us before we even know that we have a problem. Trust in the divine power can become the spark that gives purpose and meaning to life. For those dealing with serious illness, trust represents a powerful catalyst that energizes healing!

Today, many have embraced the NEWSTART program around the world. With cancer especially, healthful living is crucial.

Now back to Step 2 - The Recovery Diet

As described earlier, Step 1, the Reverse Diet, is useful for a brief period of time for those whose health has been severely compromised. Step 2, the Recovery Diet may be started as soon as solid foods are desired. In addition to juices, fresh raw fruits and vegetables are encouraged, along with cooked whole foods, with the latter comprising approximately 25% of the diet. The goal is to consistently incorporate an abundance of raw vegetables and vegetable juices to flood the diseased cells with powerful healing nutrients. The following is a suggested menu, which can be altered to personal preference, for example, swapping the cooked foods from the evening to the lunch meal.

The Recovery Diet - A typical day's menu supplemented by juices and liquids between meals:

- **Upon arising** – water or miso broth or herb tea with fresh squeezed lemon juice
  Fresh fruit or fruit smoothie or fresh fruit juice with green powder / liquid supplement
- **Breakfast** – Whole grain cooked cereal with organic non-dairy milk (soy, almond, hemp)
- Fresh vegetable juice, 2 cups
- **Lunch** – Soup (raw or cooked),
  Vegetable salad with raw seeds, raw nuts, and nutritional food yeast (not rising yeast used in baking)
- Fresh vegetable juice, 2 cups
- Water or miso broth or herb tea
- Fresh vegetable juice, 2 cups
- **Supper** – Baked sweet potato, brown rice, or other whole grains
  Steamed vegetables
  Raw vegetable salad

Remember, a good nutritional program is an integral part for recovery; because it takes time for the body to rebuild and recover. Stay with this powerful nutritional plan to enhance the body's self-healing process. Be assured that you are not only providing the best nutrients but also supporting the whole system with healing energy from natural therapies including exercises, the use of water, sunlight, temperance, fresh air, adequate rest, and trust in God. This lifestyle is not just a temporary fix but a permanent part of a healthy life. Recovery can be realized when one follows a consistent NEWSTART lifestyle every day.

CHAPTER 15

THE RIGHT DIET

The Right Diet benefits everyone because it is a plant-based whole foods diet, low in fat, and high in healthy nutrients. Research has shown that plant-based foods lower the risk for cancer by 60 to 80 percent through diet alone. We can reduce our risk for cancer by eating plant-based whole foods. They provide phytonutrients with powerful antioxidants and anti-inflammatory compounds to protect us from cancer. Plant foods also contain fiber which soaks up toxins, chemicals, cholesterol, drugs, and other wastes to eliminate them from the body. A diet with an abundance of beans, grains, fruits and vegetables is the *right diet*, particularly with inclusion of more raw foods which contain cancer-fighting elements.

Why do we need to consume more raw foods?

The raw fruits, raw vegetables, sprouted grains and beans contain valuable life force or vital energy known as enzymes. For superior health, the Right Diet should be about 50 to 75 per cent raw.

What are enzymes? Enzymes are the "labor force" of the body.[1] Like spark plugs that make cars run, enzymes are needed for every chemical action and reaction in the human body. In addition to enabling digestion and absorption of food, they also aid in detoxification, breakdown of blood clots, and protection of our immune system.

More importantly, enzymes can even digest cancers by penetrating the protective coverings of cancer cells.[2] It appears that enzymes dissolve the fibrin coating of cancer cells, which then allows the body's defense mechanisms to work more efficiently. In earlier chapters (Chapters 1, 5) we talked about the enzymes' ability to remove the camouflage coating on the surfaces of cancer cells when our body has adequate enzyme storage. But this storage can become depleted. How so?

At birth, we are given an enzyme reserve which I call our "enzyme bank account." But this reserve can become depleted by stress, aging, and a diet high in processed cooked foods. However, consumption of more enzyme rich foods will deposit enzymes back into the bank. But similarly to our checking account, there is a danger that we may overdraw our reserves resulting in insufficient funds.

Enzymes are heat sensitive. At temperatures above 118°F, enzymes begin to lose their full potential work energy; above 120°F they become sluggish; and over 130°F they die. They are also rendered lifeless through heat processing such as canning, microwaving, and pasteurization. But eating food in the raw and living state nourishes the cells and tissues efficiently and quickly. There is no substitute for live foods to nourish, to regenerate, and to rebuild a sick body back to health.

However, some foods need to be cooked. Certain grains and legumes require cooking to inactivate the phytates from blocking mineral absorption and trypsin inhibitors from hampering protein digestion. Cooking, soaking, or sprouting the grains and legumes will help to destroy these phytates and trypsin inhibitors.

The Right Diet menu

The Right Diet is comprised of unprocessed whole beans, whole grains, fruits, and vegetables, approximately 50 – 75% of which would ideally be raw and prepared without fat.

- **Upon arising** – Water or miso broth or herb tea with freshly squeezed lemon juice
  Fresh fruit juice with green powder / liquid supplement or fruit smoothie or fresh whole fruit
- **Breakfast** – whole grain cereal with non-dairy organic milk (soy, almond, hemp) or other breakfast items as desired
- Fresh vegetable juice, 2 cups

- **Lunch** – Burritos or Burger or Wraps or Soups or Stews
  Vegetable salad with avocados, raw seeds, raw nuts, nutritional food yeast
- Fresh vegetable juice, 2 cups
- Water or miso broth or herb tea
- **Supper** – Casserole or pasta with vegetables or baked potato or sweet potato, brown rice and beans or other whole grains
  Steamed vegetables
  Raw vegetable salad

Again, this is a suggested menu. One may adjust to suit one's own eating preference and schedule. As a reminder, always drink the juices on an empty stomach, between meals for maximum absorption.

Foods to Include:

The Right Diet includes all unprocessed, unrefined whole plant-based foods without chemical additives, and preferably organically grown.

Fruits – all kinds of fresh, tree ripened, frozen, canned without sugar, unsulfured dried fruit

Vegetables – all kinds of fresh, frozen and canned without sugar, all varieties of sprouts, herbs, potatoes, yams, sweet potatoes and other root vegetables

Whole Grains – whole wheat, buckwheat, whole oats, rye, barley, millet, quinoa, amaranth, spelt, faro, whole rice (brown, black, red, wild), sorghum grains, teff, and a variety of whole grain breads, pastas, noodles, and many other whole grain products. Although couscous is made from durum wheat milled to remove bran and germ, it adds a nice addition to the menu. Durum wheat is a variety of triticum turgidum, hard wheat with high protein content.

Beans and Legumes – all types dried beans such as soy, black, red, pink, pinto, red kidney, lima, adzuki, fava, mung beans and white beans (cannellini – large Italian kidney, great northern, and navy). Other types include lentils (red, brown, green), split peas, garbanzos (chickpeas), and many sprouted beans. Also included are products made from the beans and grains such as tofu, seitan, tempeh and veggie burgers. Always read the labels and avoid refined oils, fats, sugars, and chemical additives.

Nuts and Seeds – all raw, unprocessed, and raw nut butters without refined sugars and oils.

Beverages – purified filtered water, freshly extracted vegetable juices, fresh squeezed fruit juices, caffeine-free herbal teas, caffeine-free green tea, cereal-based beverages, whole soy coffee (see recipe), and non-dairy milk (almond, soy, cashew, hemp, rice), and fresh fruit and vegetable smoothies

Sweeteners – all raw, unrefined, unprocessed whole natural sweeteners (Rapadura, Sucanat, Turbinado), organic agave nectar, stevia, raw unfiltered honey, pure maple syrup, brown rice syrup, sorghum molasses, barely malt syrup, black strap molasses, coconut palm sugar (from coconut flower blossom nectar), carob powder, date sugar. Just remember that these unrefined sugars are *concentrated* foods, so do limit the amount and frequency of use.

Foods to Avoid:

All commercially processed and prepared canned, packaged, bottled, boxed, wrapped products containing animal foods (meat, poultry, fish, seafood,) milk, dairy products, eggs, refined sugars, artificial sweeteners, refined fats, oils, and chemical additives.

Animal foods – meat, poultry, fish, seafood

Milk, dairy products; and milk and dairy containing products

Eggs and egg containing products

Beverages – alcohol, coffee, caffeinated drinks, sodas, soft drinks, sport drinks, sweetened juices.

Sugars and sweets – all refined, white or brown sugar (brown sugar is actually white sugar with added molasses for color), high fructose corn syrup, corn syrup, palm sugar, candies, chocolates, and commercially prepared baked goods and products containing refined sugars and artificial sweeteners.

Artificial sweeteners and chemical additives – all synthetic sweeteners, artificial colors, artificial flavors, GMOs, preservatives, and additives found in most commercial foods and beverages.

Seasonings – Monosodium glutamate (MSG) and related spices are used in food to enhance flavor. MSG is found in almost all processed or manufactured food. Unless a product contains 99 percent free glutamic acid, manufacturers are not required by FDA to label it as MSG. The products with less than 99 percent pure MSG are called by disguised names: hydrolyzed vegetable protein, plant protein, sodium caseinate, calcium caseinate, yeast extract, textured protein, flavoring, natural flavoring, natural beef or chicken flavoring, spices, carrageenan, enzymes, soy protein concentrate, whey protein, and bouillon, broth, and stock containing MSG.

Salad dressings, soups and dips – all commercially prepared with dairy products, eggs, refined oils, sugar, preservatives, and chemical additives.

Refined grains and beans– all refined, white flour and white flour products (noodles, pasta, breads, pastries, crackers, cold breakfast cereals, chips, pretzels, and baked products); white rice; and other refined grains and refined beans plus many products made from them.

Refined fats and oils and snacks – including all manufactured products containing refined fats, trans fats, hydrogenated oils found in mixes, gravies, prepared entrees, crackers, chips, plus many snacks, and other packaged items.

Eat more cancer fighting foods

In the following section I have listed some specific foods that one needs to include frequently. They have powerful cancer fighting properties to further enhance the body's innate ability to heal.

1. Eat Greens and Cruciferous Veggies – Leafy greens and cruciferous vegetables such as spinach, cabbage, kale, chards, collards, broccoli, broccoli sprouts, Brussels sprouts, bok choy, cauliflower, arugulas, watercress, and many other greens. These all contain natural compounds (sulforaphane and indole-3-carbinols) that can detoxify carcinogens, increase the body's natural killer cells against tumors, promote suicide of cancer cells (apoptosis), and decrease the risk of metastases.[3,4] That's the "phyto" power in vegetables.

Frequent consumption of the cruciferous vegetables can lower cancer risks and increase survival.[5] However, one caveat – certain active components are destroyed by *overcooking*. Just remember to incorporate more raw greens and cruciferous vegetables every day. Let me explain why.

Eating fruits and vegetables can change genes: Is it possible that eating fruits and vegetables can alter genes? Yes. For example:

9p21 gene – Researchers reported that those consuming generous amounts of fruits and vegetables can modify the gene designated as 9p21, which is the strongest marker for heart disease. People with the 9p21 gene increase their risk for heart disease. Those who lowered their risk ate at least 2 servings of fruits and vegetables per day. But, eating *raw* fruits and vegetables showed the most impact! It appears one can indeed turn off a bad gene by consuming a healthy diet with plenty of raw fruits and vegetables.[6] That's "phyto" power in raw fruits and vegetables!

p53 gene – In Chapter 14, we talked about the p53 gene that regulates the cell cycle. Another important function is that p53 prevents mutation by protecting cells from becoming cancerous.[7] When p53 is intact, the human system can automatically initiate its own repair, or if damage is beyond repair, it can induce cell death. But when p53 itself is damaged, tumors can develop. The p53 gene is damaged by chemicals, radiation, viruses, and certain foods such as carcinogens in fried foods, animal products, and sugary foods. Lack of rest and insufficient sleep can also injure p53. The damaged p53 gene, however, can revert back to normal, as found by researchers.[8] It has been shown that high doses of beta-carotene can transform the p53 back to normal gene. Beta-carotene is abundant in colorful fruits and vegetables. People have recovered from cancer by drinking the juices of colorful fresh fruits and vegetables.[9]

2. Eat Colors – Colorful fruits and vegetables are loaded with protective phytonutrients. It appears that the deeper the color, the more vitamins, minerals and phytonutrients they have.[10] Presently there are over 4,000 known plant pigments (flavonoids) in our food, plus many more unknown and unnamed ones.

Colorful fruits and vegetables are rich in thousands of flavonoids and hundreds of carotenoids and anthocyanins. These powerful compounds can stimulate immune cells to attack tumor cells, inhibit cancer cell growth, promote cancer cell death (apoptosis), and block metastases.

Among the top fruits and vegetables are carrots, spinach, kale, broccoli, Brussels sprouts, collards, chards, asparagus, bell peppers, zucchini, squash, sweet potatoes, yams, purple yams, purple cauliflower, eggplants, tomatoes, watermelon, beets, apples, cherries, pink grapefruit, grapes, figs, papayas, pineapples, other citrus fruits, apricots, persimmons, plums, pomegranates, and a variety of berries, plus common herbs such as parsley, rosemary, thyme, oregano, basil and mint.

The superiority of berries merits special mention. They contain cancer-fighting antioxidants, one of the most powerful being anthocyanosides. Blueberries and black raspberries have high concentrations of anthocyanins. These phytochemicals are known to slow the growth of premalignant cells, and prevent new blood vessels from forming that can feed and spread cancerous tumors (Chapter 1).[11]

Another fruit having strong antioxidant activity is the pomegranate. Its anti-inflammatory substances such as tannins and anthocyanins and its ability to inhibit tumor growth and increase tumor cell death make it highly valuable. Studies from several universities have shown pomegranates contain cancer-fighting properties against prostate, breast, lung, and colon cancers.[12,13]

Clinical trials in men with prostate cancer showed that drinking 8 oz. of pomegranate juice a day significantly slowed tumor growth and had a chemotherapeutic effect on tumor cells.[14]

3. Eat Soy and Other Dried Beans – Soy beans contain anti-carcinogenic properties. In animal experiments, soybeans can reduce mammary cancers.[15] The isoflavones in the soybeans can prevent tumor development and slow tumor growth.[16] Containing plant-estrogens that can block the stimulation of cancer cells by sex hormones (estrogens and testosterones), they provide protection from prostate, uterine, breast, and ovarian cancers.[17] Whole soy bean products such as soy milk, soy yogurt, tofu, tempeh, and miso are preferable to their derivatives that appear in refined, processed, texturized form.

All dried beans, particularly the deep colored red beans and black beans, are rich in protein, B vitamins, minerals and fiber, providing an abundant supply of antioxidants and bioflavonoids that protect against colon and breast cancer.[11]

4. Eat Pungent Vegetables and Spices – Garlic, onions, leeks, shallots, and chives contain sulfur compounds that are important in reducing the risk for breast, prostate, lung, skin, and colon cancer.[17] Both garlic and onions are believed to block the formation of nitrosamines – potent carcinogens that can form in the stomach. Researchers found that death rates from stomach cancer were 10 times lower in a county in China where residents consumed large amounts of garlic as compared to a nearby county where the diet did not contain garlic. In Italy, researchers also found those who ate garlic and onions regularly had less than half the normal risk of developing stomach cancer. The Iowa Women's Health Study found those who consumed highest quantities of garlic had a 50 percent lower risk of colon cancers than women who ate the least.[11]

Capsaicin, the compound responsible for pungency found in chilies, can kill cancerous cells without hurting healthy cells. Studies show that capsaicin inhibits the proliferation of cancerous cells in the lungs, pancreas, and prostate. Mexicans who smoke but eat chili peppers had a relatively low rate of lung cancer.[18]

Other spices include ginger and turmeric. Curcumin is a component of turmeric that can activate the immune functions, and down regulate pro-inflammatory chemicals. Both ginger and turmeric can counter act the inflammatory processes.[19]

5. Eat Lignans – Lignans is a type of fiber found in flaxseeds and black sesame seeds. Small amounts also appear in other seeds, whole grains, legumes, fruits and vegetables. Diets high in lignan-rich foods have been associated with lower incidence of prostate cancer, breast, ovarian and uterine cancers. Include some seeds daily.

6. Eat Fiber – A high intake of dietary fiber such as cereal fiber and whole grains was associated with a reduced risk of colorectal cancer.[20] Fiber also helps the body to remove excess hormones that contribute to cancer, particularly to hormone related breast cancer. Vegetarians showed significantly decreased estrogen production. At the same time, vegetarians showed a greater removal of excess and unneeded hormones when compared with omnivores.[21] It appears that a vegetarian diets helps to expel cancer-causing hormones, along with carcinogens and other toxic compounds from the body.[22]

7. Eat Seeds – Seeds support life. Particularly important are the nitrilosides in edible seeds, grains, fruits, and vegetables. Any food containing seeds has nitrilosides, such as millet, tomatoes, cucumbers, eggplants, peppers, zucchini, berries, figs, sunflower seeds, sesame seeds, pumpkin seeds, and flaxseeds.

8. Include Mushrooms and Seaweeds – They have pronounced benefit on the immune system by slowing cancer growth and causing cancer cell death. Reshi, shiitake, and maitake mushrooms contain a substance called 1,3-beta-glucan which can slow the growth of tumors in animals. White button mushrooms also contain the important antioxidant selenium which lowers the risk for stomach, lung, colon, and prostate cancers.[17] Naturally low in fact, mushrooms and seaweeds provide high-quality protein, deliver more minerals than many meats, are rich in the B vitamins and some vitamin D.

9. Green Tea – Green tea contains polyphenols which reduces the growth of new vessels needed for tumor growth and metastases. Green tea is a powerful antioxidant, detoxifier and cancer cell killer. Decaffeinated green tea is recommended.

10. Super Green Foods – They are truly *super* because they are *living foods* that contain antitumor nutrients. They can help repair diseased cells, mitigate toxicity, neutralize pollutants and free radicals, oxygenate the blood, and interfere with the action of carcinogens.[23] This powerful group includes algae, spirulina, chlorella, alfalfa, wheat grass, barley grass, and other cereal grasses.

These cancer fighters are part of a plant-based unprocessed whole foods diet. Eating a handful of blueberries over ice cream cannot fight cancer; or a tofu burger wash down with a can of soda; or even a glass of carrot juice with steak! But rather, a plant-based whole foods diet with extra helpings of cancer fighter foods can be powerful ammunition against cancers.

The Right Diet a Part of Daily Life

The person with cancer needs to incorporate the Right Diet as a way of life. From clinical observations, we have noticed recurrences of cancers often within a few months when animal foods were consumed again. Some recurrences may take longer. When the doctor declares a patient to be cancer free, this could lead to a false supposition that one is free to eat anything. Often people will resume consumption of dairy, eggs, and animal foods, thinking that "a little bit won't hurt." Well-meaning friends and family may encourage a wider selection of foods, but resisting the urge to return to the old, disease-inducing diet will reap continued health.

I want to emphasize that it is of crucial importance that the Right Diet, a plant-based unprocessed whole foods, be conscientiously followed and maintained for life. It has been found that continuing the 100% change in diet for as little as 28 days allows the taste buds to discover new and exciting tastes and the body to enjoy subsequent improved health. Make it a "permanent-fad," not a "temporary fix."

First, avoid **RATS** - foods that promote cancer:

> *__R__efined grains, beans, fats, oils*
> *__A__nimal foods including milk, dairy, and eggs*
> *__T__oxic additives, chemicals, flavor enhancers, GMOs*
> *__S__ugars all refined*

Second, include **BGFVs** (___BIG FAVOR___) - foods that fight cancer:

> *__B__eans*
> *__G__rains*
> *__F__ruits*
> *__V__egetables*

141

CHAPTER 16

WHY BUY ORGANIC?

In spite of the complexity of the cancer saga, simply put, toxicity contributes to cancer, whether from food, environment or lifestyle habits. To prevent and to recover from cancer, one needs to reduce the toxic load in the body. By consuming organic foods, we assist the body in lowering its toxicity burden.

On Mother's Day this year, I received an unusual gift from our daughter Shari and granddaughter Kyra. They took us out to visit an organic farm. I did not expect to see the enormous cultivated land with vegetables, berries and fruit trees spread out as far as the eyes can see. Tour guides took us on the flatbed trucks to view their vast gardens. We could pick any vegetables, berries, and stuff them into the bags the farm provided. We competed with who can stuff the most and the largest sweet onions, kale, cauliflower, strawberries among many others into our bulging bags! Finally the guides escorted us up on a grassy hill overlooking the valley covered with thousands of rows of organic edible plants. Under a beautiful canopy we were invited to tables where cool water and freshly picked vegetables were served. That day the chef prepared sautéed sweet onions and zucchini, freshly picked just that morning. What an attractive and flavorful treat for our taste buds!

In organic farming the soil is nurtured by using only organic matter, rotating crops, and planting beneficial cover crops. Conventional farming uses toxic chemicals and synthetic additives. Over half of Americans actually prefer organic foods. Some choose organic to support local farms and others want to avoid toxins in conventionally grown products.[1]

Organic foods are not only less toxic, but they are superior in nutritional value. A European study finds that organic produce has up to 40% more antioxidants than their conventional counterparts.[2]

Conversely, conventional farming causes plants to produce fewer phytochemicals. Studies have demonstrated that phytochemicals in edible plants can prevent and reverse every human ailment known, from Alzheimer's, to cancers to cardiovascular and other chronic diseases. The greatest advantage of organic fruits and vegetables is that they contain more protective phytonutrients than do chemically grown crops.[3]

Unfortunately, organic foods do cost more. Take time to read labels and look for the following:

1. "USDA Organic" seal means that the product is free from synthetic ingredients and toxic pesticides.
2. "Organic" indicates that the product contains at least 95% organic ingredients.
3. "Made with organic ingredients" means that the product has a minimum of 70% organic ingredients but is not eligible to carry an organic seal.[4]

What do the sticker numbers mean on the produce?

You will notice on the produce stickers a "PLU" followed with numbers. PLU means Price Look Up code. These code numbers are used by the cashiers at the check-out counter. For the consumers, the PLU numbers tell us pertinent information:

1. PLU stickers with four digits beginning with a "3" or "4" means that the produce is conventionally grown. It has been sprayed with weed killers and chemical pesticides.
2. PLU stickers with five digits beginning with "8" indicate that this item is genetically engineered with genes that have been manipulated (altered) to produce a larger and brighter colored food. They may also have been chemically treated.
3. PLU stickers with five digits beginning with "9" means that this produce was raised organically and was not treated with any chemicals.[5]

Remember to read the "PLU" numbers carefully on labels:
    Organic – starts with 9
    Conventional – starts with 3 or 4
    Genetically modified – starts with 8

Which produce contains the most and the least amounts of pesticides?

The researchers at the Environmental Working Group analyzed 89,000 produce for pesticide contents. Their tests determined the most contaminated fruits and vegetables by the number of toxic chemicals. Celery topped the chart because the stalks are very porous, which retain the most pesticides.[6] Those fruits and vegetables containing higher pesticide residue should be avoided and replaced by organic ones. Those with lower pesticide levels are safer and the conventionally grown may be purchased. But clean well with organic vegetable and fruit wash. Take a look at the latest findings listed below:

Lowest pesticide levels - least contaminated:

Asparagus, avocados, bananas, cantaloupe (domestic), cabbage, eggplant, grapefruit, kiwi, mangoes, mushrooms, onions, pineapples, sweet corn, sweet peas, sweet potatoes, watermelon.[7]

Highest pesticide levels - Buy these organic:

Apples, bell peppers, blueberries, celery, cherries, grapes, kale, collard greens, lettuce, nectarines, peaches, pears, potatoes, red raspberries, spinach, strawberries.[7]

We need to be selective. Nearly seven out of ten items on the store shelves contain ingredients that have been genetically modified. Take time to read the stickers on the fruits and the vegetables.

More Tips:

1. Shop at local farmers' markets for organic and freshest produce.

2. Buy organic fruits and vegetables in season or get organic frozen and organic canned products. Read labels to avoid refined sugars and oils.

3. Plant an organic garden using organic soil and organic fertilizers. Even in small areas, you can grow vegetables in pots and containers.

4. Grow your own sprouts and wheat grass in the kitchen.

CHAPTER 17

CONCLUSION

In this book we have presented the most advanced, the safest, the most non-invasive, and the most effective therapy to prevent, arrest, and reverse cancer. We like to consider phytotherapy as the "grand prix" of cancer therapy!

Irrefutable evidence abounds regarding the multi-functions of phytotherapy: as immunotherapy, non-toxic chemotherapy, and non-surgical surgery. Due to its triple action against cancer, phyotherapy becomes a powerful armament that destroys the bad and defends the good.

First, phytotherapy is a powerful *immunotherapy* in that phytochemicals in a plant-based diet enhance the functions of macrophages, natural killer cells, and T lymphocytes. These immune cells can effectively fight all kinds of cancer, which have been documented with our own research presented in Chapters 1, 2, and 5.

Second, phytotherapy is actually an authentic, original prototype of *chemotherapy*. Many patented chemotherapeutic drugs are derived from plants, but because they have been extracted, purified and fractionated (so that they can be patented), they are extremely toxic (Chapters 2 and 6). Consequently, pain and suffering accompany chemotherapy. On the other hand, a plant-based diet contains many phytochemicals that are selectively toxic to cancer cells, and nontoxic (actually nutritive) to normal cells (Chapters 2, 3, 7). That is:

- ✓ Phytochemicals *kill* only cancer cells.
- ✓ Phytochemicals *nourish* normal cells.

This is "selectivity" at its best! Yet without side effects! Today's typical diet contains minimal phytochemicals. Instead, our diet comprises mostly animal foods, high in fats, high in sugars, and highly processed. Sadly, this type of foods produces negative effects as they feed cancer cells and starve normal cells. The first thing a cancer patient must do is to *stop eating all animal products and processed foods* which are cancer promoters.

Third, phytotherapy is *non-surgical surgery*. We have observed that cancers and tumors fall off on a strictly plant-based diet (Chapters 2, 7). Thus, phytotherapy is a natural surgery without a scalpel.

Finally, for those who are inclined to accept and believe in the teachings of the Holy Bible, we would like to share with you two health secrets from the Bible.

1. The plant-based diet was ordained by our Creator from the dawn of earth's history as recorded in the first book of the Bible, Genesis 1: 29. The original diet consisted of grains, fruits, nuts, and seeds. The early inhabitants lived to nearly 1000 years without any diseases, let alone cancer. When animal foods were introduced, the average life span plummeted to 150 years. As more animal foods were consumed in place of a plant-based diet, human lifespan continued to dwindle to the present time of 70 to 80 years. Now scientific research has affirmed that to stay away from cancer and other deadly diseases, we need to return to the diet God originally ordained, namely, a plant-based diet.

2. In the last book of the Bible, Revelation 18:23-24, God foretold that Satan would use sorceries to deceive the people in all nations. The word "sorceries" in Greek (the original language of New Testament of the Bible) is "*farmakeia*" or pharmacy/drugs in English. In other words, the Bible warns us against the use of drugs; raising the possibility that their use can further impede the chances for a person to recover from cancer. Perhaps a reevaluation of the current therapies needs to also include phytotherapy. The good news is that we can stop cancer when we choose to follow the biblical injunctions because any sustainable cure requires a strong immune system supported by wholesome foods and a healthy lifestyle.

Simple Solutions in a Nutshell: If you have cancer or someone you know of has cancer, here are some steps you may wish to incorporate immediately:

1. Stop eating all animal products and processed foods, as they promote cancer growth.
2. Eat a plant-based diet with its thousands of phytochemicals that destroy cancer cells and strengthen immune cells.
3. Go to sleep every night before 10 pm.
4. If the tumor is small, sit tight. If the tumor is large, you may opt to have it removed with conventional methods.
5. If it is too difficult for you to do it on your own, you may consider spending some time in a wellness center to learn how to change your diet and lifestyle habits (see appendix).

Take time to consider all options. Do not rush into any hasty decisions. A cancer diagnosis can be an impetus towards healthier living in which one can experience the best years yet to come. This has been the experience of thousands who are a living monument, demonstrating the value of phytotherapy in effectively stopping cancer. We are awed and inspired by these men, women, and children once ravaged with cancer who are now enjoying a healthy, vibrant life. We share in their joy. Our wish for you is that you too may experience a healthy, productive, cancer-free life! Thank you for journeying with us. *God Bless! Bon Voyage!*

STOP CANCER right now
This is how
Go enjoy the world outside,
It's good for you
and the whole world wide.
If you eat unhealthy it will make you small
Eat good and get strong and tall.
God blesses you every day He's going to say,
"Just be you and who you are
You are a wonderful star."

Kyra Kaya, 8 years old

Kyra Kaya,
THE THIRD AUTHOR

Kyra wrote these poems when she was in the second grade. One morning after being dropped off by her parents on their way to work, eight-year old Kyra was waiting for her car pool ride to school blurted out:

"Grandma, how's your book coming along?"
"Oh, I'm still working on it," I replied.
"May I write some poems for your book?" Kyra asked
"Sure."

Within 5 minutes, Kyra composed the three poems appear in the beginning, middle and at the end of this book just before the car pulled up.

Here lie the keys on how to STOP CANCER through the eyes of an eight year old!

RECIPES FOR LIFE

Recipes for Life are designed with you in mind. My recipes differ from most other recipes because I use only ingredients from whole unprocessed foods. These recipes use food as "medicine."

Not all plant-based or vegan foods can be considered healthy. In fact some can be classified as "junk" foods. When you go to the supermarket, you will find more vegan products than ever before, but we need to know "what's in there." Many of them contain refined sugars, bleached flour, trans fats, refined oils, artificial colors, synthetic sweeteners, flavor enhancers, chemical preservatives plus toxic additives. Be sure to read labels before you buy.

Recently some of our relatives and friends have switched to an all plant-based whole foods diet. The results not only benefited those individuals, but also the rest of the family.

Few months ago, my nephew Brian made the drastic switch to an all plant-based diet! Over 20 years ago when in middle school, he spent some time in the author's lab studying garlic for his science project. As a result, he captured the grand prize in the Tennessee State Science and Engineering fair for his research on garlic. Based on his research, the then 12-year-old Brian boldly concluded that "Garlic cures cancer." Now even toddlers begin to pick up trendy vocabulary. Although somewhat oblivious to the ongoing dietary changes in their home, Brian's three-year-old daughter Caitlin picked up a newly acquired word – vegan. One day after church a Korean lady asked, "Are you Korean?" to which Caitlin replied in all seriousness, "No, I'm not Korean. I'm vegan!"

This section of the book, Recipes for Life, focuses on the functional components found in unprocessed whole plant-based foods. That is, I select ingredients for their beneficial healing properties. By consuming a plant-based diet of unrefined whole foods without refined sugars or chemical additives and low in fat, one can minimize the risk of all killer diseases. Because of their naturally occurring "medicinal" values, I wish to encourage everyone to consume more plant-based whole foods every day.

Many recipes were developed in my kitchen and taste-tested by family members and friends. Recipes from others were modified to meet my criteria that include only unprocessed whole foods with minimum of partially refined ingredients. Even healthy ingredients (e.g. natural sweeteners, raw nuts) are greatly reduced in the recipes. I recommend the use of unrefined sweeteners, unprocessed sea salt and preferably organic ingredients.

Whenever a recipe calls for "frying" or "sautéing" remember, no oil or fat is used. Instead, I use a little water or broth as oil. A good heavy stainless steel pan or a non-stick Green Pan works well for "frying." There are safe non-stick non-toxic pans that brown foods evenly.

In addition, I have provided nutritional tips with each recipe; hopefully, this will encourage you to try them. Have fun experimenting and improving my recipes. I appreciate your input.

SMOOTHIES AND JUICES

Basic Breakfast Green Smoothie
Power Breakfast Smoothie
Basic Carrot Juice Plus
All Greens Drink
Carrot, Beet, and Cucumber Juice (CBC)
Carrot, Kale, and Parsley Juice (CKP)

Basic Breakfast Green Smoothie

2 fresh or frozen bananas
2 T green powder or handful of kale, spinach or other greens
2 soft dates
1½ cups water

Process all ingredients in a blender till smooth. Enjoy.

We have been drinking this breakfast green smoothie for nearly three decades! From this basic drink, you can add any fresh organic fruit in season; then just omit the dates. For those wishing to increase the calories, you can add some soaked almonds, walnuts or just put in one tablespoon of raw almond butter and or ½ avocado.

I consider algae (spirulina, chlorella, blue-green algae), wheatgrass, barley grass, alfalfa, and other greens as super foods. They are nutrient dense containing all the nutritional complexes, micro nutrients and trace elements plus thousands of unnamed phytonutrients that speed up recovery and keep us energized. The green powder (or liquid) enhances the body's immune system and has anti-tumor and anti-cancer properties. The green smoothie is easily assimilated, and also serves as a powerful daily detoxifier.

If you have aloe vera plant, you can put it into the smoothie (just scrap off the sharp pin-like needles along the sides of the leaf). Its detoxification properties can help remove heavy metals and other contaminates out of the body.

Power Breakfast Smoothie

1 ripe banana
1–2 other fruit (any fresh in season or frozen)
2 T Hemp Protein (raw cold milled organic hemp protein powder)
2 T green powder
1 T raw organic almond butter
1 ½ – 2 c water

Process all ingredients in a blender until smooth.

Walking with two neighbor ladies one early morning; they wanted to know what I eat and where I get "all that energy." "Where do you get your protein?" and "What are you going to eat for breakfast this morning?" I told them to try this Power Breakfast Smoothie. Pack with nutrients, hemp protein provides a balance of amino acids, essential fatty acids and valuable fiber. When combined with fresh fruit, nutrient-rich green powder, the Power Breakfast Smoothie furnishes a power breakfast unparalleled to none!

Nutritionally, I consider the almond as the "king" among nuts. Almonds' antioxidants protect our cells from damage by free radicals and maintain the integrity and health of the cells. Almonds furnish one of the best sources of vitamin E which may reduce the risk of cancer and heart disease.

Basic Carrot Juice Plus

5 lbs. organic carrots
3 organic apples
Hand full of organic greens and or other vegetables

1. Put through a vegetable juicer that separates the pulp from the juice. This makes approximately 6 cups of juice.
2. Store juice in glass jars with lids in the refrigerator. Use within 2 days.

You can add any vegetables (spinach, kale, beet greens, collards, chard, dandelion, lettuce, cucumbers, celery, summer squash, bell peppers, parsley) to the Basic Carrot Juice Plus.

I consider fresh carrot juice as the king of vegetable juices. Its unique synergy of enzymes, vitamins, minerals and flavonoids provides a fast-delivery system to our bodies. It boosts the immune system, slows down the aging process, reduces the risk of cancer, protects the cardiovascular system, and improves digestion. Carrots have powerful cleansing properties in detoxifying the liver and reduce toxicity of the blood.

All Greens Drink

Handful organic kale leaves
1 organic cucumber
1 leaf organic Swiss chard, optional
1 stalk organic celery
1 organic green apple

Put through vegetable juicer. Roll up the green leaves in a "ball," push through with firm celery and apples. This will make it easier to go through the juicer. Enjoy immediately.

The kale, cucumber, Swiss chard (if using) in combination with celery and tart apple make a delightful refreshing drink. Instead of kale, one can use spinach, collards, broccoli, cilantro, cabbage or any other greens. You can also add a tiny piece of fresh ginger.

This drink is so rich in nutrients that no bottled synthetic supplements can compete. Because of the absence of fiber, this drink delivers maximum nutrient with near-immediate absorption of vitamins and minerals to heal the body.

Carrot, Beet, and Cucumber Juice (CBC)

1 lb. carrots
1 beet and handful beet leaves
1–2 cucumbers

Process all vegetables in the juicer. Enjoy.

The CBC (Carrot, Beet and Cucumber) Juice is truly a body builder. These vegetables can correct an acidic (toxic) condition often the result of consuming too much meat, refined food and sugars. Their nutrients will benefit those with anemia, high blood pressure, kidney and gall stones, liver problems, and inflammation of kidneys, lungs, and bladder.

Beet juice provides many health benefits because of its rich minerals and trace minerals. Beets are organic cleansers that can prevent the formation of cancerous tumors. The juice can also benefit those with heart attacks and strokes. However, a word of caution – beet juice should not be taken alone. Because of its cleansing effect, one may feel a little dizzy if taken too much at a time. Only drink no more than 2 ounces at a time; preferably with other juices. Or you can dilute with more water.

Cucumber is one of the best natural diuretic vegetable that helps in promoting the flow of urine. Cucumbers are rich in silicon and sulfur both can promote healthy hair, nail and skin.

Carrot, Kale, and Parsley Juice (CKP)

5 lbs. organic carrots
1 bunch organic kale, use center ribs only (save leaves for salad)
½ bunch organic parsley, leaves and stems

Process all vegetables in the juicer. This recipe yields approximately 6 cups of juice.

The Carrot, Kale and Parsley Juice (CKP) is filled with the best nutrition that nature offers. Some consider carrot juice as "liquid gold." Carrot juice is one of the most healing foods. Drinking a glass of carrot juice daily will do much more for us than taking bottles of supplements. Just eating one carrot a day significantly reduces cancer risks. It also boosts the immune system.

Kale is called "the new beef," because of its high iron content. Per calorie, kale has more iron than beef. Iron is essential for the formation of hemoglobin and enzymes; and for transporting oxygen throughout the body.

I like to dub kale as the "new green cow!" Better yet, kale juice is the "new green milk!" Yes, per calorie, kale has more calcium than cow's milk. Kale offers organic iron and organic calcium that is easily assimilated by our body. In fact, cow's milk contains very little iron. Kale provides much vitamin K - just one cup of kale furnishes 1,327 percent of your daily need! This vitamin helps to protect us against various cancers. Furthermore, vitamin K is necessary for bone health, prevents blood clotting, and benefits people with Alzheimer's disease.

Parsley has high concentration of antioxidants which help neutralize the cancer-causing compounds. Parsley also contains immune-enhancing compounds making it an extraordinary immunity booster. Drinking parsley juice can increase the hemoglobin count. Do not drink too much parsley juice alone at one time because it is very concentrated – one or two ounces are enough. But when combined with other vegetables one can drink more.

BREAKFAST

Cooked Steel Cut Oats
Raw Granola
Oat - Wheat - Corn Mini Pancakes
Quinoa and Barley Pancakes
Basic Almond Nut Milk
Whole Soy Coffee

Cooked Steel Cut Oats

1 c steel cut oats
3 c water (or rice, soy, or nut milk)
5 pitted dates

1. Put all ingredients in a sauce pan with cover. Bring to boil.
2. Reduce heat to low. Cook approximately 15 minutes or until thickened to desired consistency. If too thick, add more liquid.

This is a crunchy and creamy cooked cereal especially welcome on a cold winter morning. I personally enjoy using dates as a natural sweetener; but you can use raisins; and add some nuts and seeds for a hearty breakfast.

Steel cut oats contain both the soluble fiber and insoluble fiber which combats cancer, lowers cholesterol, controls blood sugar and prevents constipation. Whole grains are one of the best sources of furnishing fiber that leads to longevity. Dates provide the B vitamins, iron, magnesium, potassium and fiber.

Raw Granola

½ c seed meal – ground sunflower, pumpkin, and flax seeds
½ c sliced almonds
½ c dates – soaked in ½ c water
1 T vanilla, alcohol free
6 c rolled oats
½ c walnuts (or pecans) – chopped
½ c hemp hearts (raw shelled hemp seeds) or ¼ c chia seeds
½ c pumpkin seeds
½ c black or brown sesame seeds
2 T flax seeds
½ c raisins
½ c coconut flakes, unsweetened
1 t cinnamon
½ c raw cashews, optional
2-3 ripe persimmons or other fruit – chopped or blend with dates*

1. To make seed meal, grind equal amounts of sunflower, pumpkin and flaxseeds separately in coffee grinder into find powder. Mix together. Set aside. (You can store the extra seed meal in a glass jar in refrigerator to sprinkle over cereals, salads, and yogurt).
2. Blend soaked dates and water in blender until smooth. Add vanilla and set aside. *You can also puree fresh fruit together with dates. Add a little water if needed to make paste.
3. Combine all dry ingredients in a large container. Add date puree and fresh fruit puree (if using). Mix well into the dry mixture.
4. Place on teflex sheets on trays in dehydrator at 118°F for approximately 6 - 8 hours or to desired crunchiness. This recipe makes 4 trays.

Enjoy the Raw Granola with soy, rice or almond milk. Or you can just use it as a topping over soy yogurt, fruit, salad, or cooked cereal. I enjoy using the low temperature dehydrator for "baking" because it will never burn; and it retains all the vital nutrients. Let me showcase a few ingredients in the Raw Granola:

Black sesame seeds contain valuable fibers that have a cholesterol lowering effect for cardiovascular health, reduce inflammation, and protect against colon cancers, and osteoporosis. Black sesame seeds are also rich in zinc, important in boosting the immune system. In addition, the seeds are an excellent source of magnesium and calcium. Just ¼ cup provides more than a cup of cow's milk! These minerals are important in regulating blood pressure, reduce headaches, and regulate sleep.

Hemp hearts are the edible insides of hemp seeds. Hemp seeds promote cellular recovery helpful for cancers, cardiovascular disease, neurodegenerative disorder, and autoimmune conditions.

Chia seeds provide vital nourishment. They are packed with protein, omega-3, antioxidants and fiber.

Pumpkin seeds contain phystosterols that lower cholesterol and protect against many cancers. The seeds reduce inflammation; and promote prostate health. Pumpkin seeds are a great source of magnesium. Half cup contains 92 percent of your daily need for magnesium, a mineral which most Americans are deficient.

Oat-Wheat-Corn Mini Pancakes

½ c rolled oats
¼ cup whole wheat pastry flour
¼ cup cornmeal
½ t baking powder
¼ t baking soda
1 ripe banana
1 c water (rice, soy or cashew nut milk)
1 t maple syrup or agave nectar
1 t apple cider vinegar

1. In a large bowl whisk together rolled oats, flour, cornmeal, baking powder and baking soda.
2. In a separate bowl, mash banana with a fork. Add water, maple syrup and vinegar.
3. Add the liquid mixture to the flour mixture. Stir until well blended. If batter appears dry, add little water as needed.
4. In a non-stick pan, pour small rounds of batter (2-3"). Cook over medium heat until top bubbles. Flip over and cook until done. Approximately 5 minutes on each side.

These mini pancakes are heavier than regular commercial pancake mixes. You can freeze them and reheat in a toaster oven.

Oats contain potent antioxidants properties and fiber that are helpful in preventing bowel cancers and cure constipation. Oats have one of the best sources of inositol (B vitamin) which is important for maintaining blood cholesterol levels.

Quinoa and Barley Pancakes

1 c soy milk, organic unsweetened
6–7 dates soak in ¼ cup water
¼ c raw cashews soak in ½ cup water
½ c cooked quinoa
½ cup barley flour
1 t baking powder
¼ t salt

1. To cook quinoa – cover 1 cup quinoa with water to soak for 5-10 minutes. Rinse with running water in a strainer to wash off the bitter coating. Put in a sauce pan with 2 cups fresh water. Bring to boil, simmer for ~18 minutes.
2. Process soy milk, soaked dates and water, soaked cashew and water in a blender until smooth. Place in a bowl. Stir in cooked quinoa. Save the remaining cooked quinoa for Quinoa and Black Bean Salad (see recipe under Salads).
3. In a separate bowl mix barley flour, baking powder and salt. Stir milk mixture into flour mixture.
4. In a non-stick skillet over medium heat pour pancake batter into desired sizes. Cook 2-3 minutes until done and flip over until golden brown color. If batter is too thick, thin with water. This recipe makes 8 3-inch-diameter pancakes.
5. Drizzle with agave nectar, if desire. Or top with any fresh fruit puree.

These pancakes are soft and moist. They freeze well. Just reheat in the toaster oven.

Soy milk is a good source of protein, containing all essential amino acids, essential fatty acids, vitamins, minerals and phytonutrients. Soy milk has no cholesterol.

Quinoa contains high quality protein. It is rich in lysine, an important amino acid for cellular repair. Quinoa also provides manganese which acts as antioxidant in the body to help get rid of cancer cells. Quinoa is pronounced "keen-wah."

Barley is rich in dietary fiber and the B vitamins. Barley is effective against diabetes, insulin resistance, stroke and certain cancers such as colon cancer.

Cashews are packed with dietary fibers, vitamins and minerals. Cashews also contain numerous health-promoting phytochemicals that help protect us from cancers.

Basic Almond Nut Milk

1 c blanched* soaked raw almonds
3 c water

1. Place blanched, soaked almonds and water in a blender.
2. Blend until smooth. Strain if desired.

The basic almond milk can be sweetened using dates, bananas, maple syrup or other natural sweeteners or any fruit in season. You can also add 1-2 t lecithin granules to make the almond milk creamier. From this basic almond milk recipe, you can make cashew nut milk or any seed milks. The cashews and seeds do not need to be blanched nor strained.

*To blanch almonds:

1. Pour boiling water over almonds.
2. When water has cooled slightly, use fingers to peel off skin by rubbing between the fingers.
3. Then soak in clean water for 2 hours or overnight.

Almonds provide an excellent source of plant protein. Almonds contain selenium, a powerful antioxidant; as well as calcium, phosphorus, magnesium, B vitamins, vitamin E and fiber.

Whole Soy Coffee

2 c non-GMO dried soy beans

1. Soak soy beans in water for 2 hours. Rinse and drain.
2. Place on tray and bake in oven at 350°F for 1 ½ to 1 ¾ hours until golden brown color. Stir to prevent burning*.
3. When cool, grind in powerful blender into fine powder. You can store soy coffee in a glass jar at room temperature.
4. For hot soy coffee, place 1-2 T of soy coffee in a mug, add hot water, stir and enjoy. You can sweeten it with stevia, honey, agave or whole unprocessed sugar to taste. There may be some soy residue at the bottom of cup, chew well for additional fiber.
   *For dark roasted soy coffee – bake at 350°F for 2-3 hours.

SOUPS

Corn Soup
Cool Tomato Soup
Cool Mushroom Soup
Pot of Beans
Butternut Squash Soup
Cool Pea Soup
Avocado and Apple Soup

Corn Soup

2 garlic – minced
¼ red onions – chopped
1 red bell pepper - chopped
1 canned (14 oz.) coconut milk
½ bag (8 oz.) frozen corn
½ t curry powder
½ cup soy milk (rice, cashew, almond or water)
½ t salt or to taste
½ c fresh cilantro, chopped as garnish

1. Put all ingredients in a saucepan over medium heat. Stir occasionally until vegetables are tender. Add salt to taste.
2. Garnish with cilantro. Enjoy.

Corn is a complex whole food that provides energy. Both garlic and onions combat cancer and are cardiovascular protective. Red bell peppers contain powerful antioxidants that resist cancer. Although a concentrated food, coconut is known to support thyroid function, and protective against free-radical damage. Turmeric, a part of curry, contains curcumin, the antioxidant that has potent anti-inflammatory affect.

There are plain coconut milk made without added chemicals. Remember, always read labels for only wholesome ingredients.

Cool Tomato Soup

4 c fresh tomatoes – diced. Save ¼ c for garnish
1 t extra virgin cold pressed olive oil
1 t agave nectar or raw honey, optional
1 ½ c water
Fresh basil leaves – chopped

1. Blend tomatoes, oil, agave nectar, and water in blender till smooth.
2. Pour soup into bowls. Garnish with tomatoes and basil leaves.

Tomatoes contain lycopene, powerful antioxidant that helps the body resist cancer and its progression. Tomatoes protect the heart and the prostate.

Cool Mushroom Soup

Marinate the following 3 items in a bowl:
2 c mushroom – sliced (button, shiitake, oyster or enoki)
1 T Bragg Liquid Aminos
1 t fresh herbs (rosemary, thyme, parsley or cilantro)

1 c raw nuts (cashews, walnuts, pecans or macadamia)
1 t extra virgin cold pressed olive oil
2 cloves garlic
2 c water
Salt to taste

1. Blend the nuts, oil, garlic and water in a blender until smooth.
2. Season with salt.
3. Pour into bowls. Garnish with marinated mushrooms and herbs.

This is a raw soup full of taste and live enzymes. In ancient Rome, mushrooms were often referred to as "Food for the gods." In America, we consume 900 million pounds of mushroom each year, mostly the white button mushrooms.

Mushrooms contain biologically active substances shown to help prevent cancerous cells from forming or recurring. Eating mushrooms regularly has been known to decrease the number of cancerous cells in the body. Mushrooms contain L-Ergothioneine- a powerful antioxidant which scavenges free radicals, and protects our cells against DNA damages.

Pecan are loaded with antioxidants which protect against cell damage and can help fight diseases like heart disease, Alzheimer's, Parkinson's, breast and prostate cancers. Eating a handful of pecans each day may be as effective at lowering LDL "bad" cholesterol as prescription medication.

Pot of Beans

1 c soy beans – soaked 6 hours or overnight
½ c of each (red beans, garbanzos, black, and white beans) soaked
1 c dehydrated soy curls or gluten – rehydrated
½ c whole kernels of wheat, oats or barley
1 potato – chopped with skin
1 carrot – chopped
1 celery stalk – chopped
1 c Napa or head cabbage – chopped
1 onion – chopped
1 c tomatoes – chopped
1 c corn – frozen or canned
1 thumb size ginger – chopped
4 cloves of garlic – chopped
2 chili peppers – chopped, optional
1 t. onion powder
1 T Bragg Liquid Aminos
½ t apple cider vinegar
Salt and herbs to taste

1. Discard soaked water and drain beans.
2. In a slow cooker or large pot, add enough fresh water to cover the soaked beans and whole grains. Cook for 6-8 hours until all beans (especially soybeans) are tender.
3. When beans are almost done, add potatoes, vegetables and seasonings; cook until tender. Adjust seasonings to taste.

The Pot of Beans is just a "pot of everything" edible that you have in your kitchen. Soybeans usually take longer to cook, so be sure they are tender before adding the vegetables Use any beans or other vegetables you have on hand.

I am a proponent of incorporating whole beans and legumes frequently in the diet. They have sustained civilizations for thousands of years due to their nutritional superiority without the cholesterol, fat and chemicals in processed foods.

Soybean is the richest plant source of protein. It contains 43 percent protein; other legumes contain 20 to 25 percent protein. Soy protein is also the highest quality equal to that of meat and milk protein. Soybeans contain omega-3 fatty acid, which helps to reduce risk of both heart disease and cancer.

Red beans contain one of the richest food sources in antioxidants. Frequent consumption of red beans helps the body fight free radicals and reduces the risk of cancer and other diseases.

Garbanzo beans provide an excellent source of soluble fiber. One cup of garbanzo beans supplies half a day's requirement for fiber. One unusual health property of garbanzo is their high molybdenum content. Molybdenum is a trace mineral that helps to detoxify sulfite, compounds which are found in many prepared food products, dried fruits, and in wine.

Black beans contain different flavonoids with enormous antioxidant potential and high content of phytochemicals. Studies show that eating black beans will reduce risk of certain cancers.

White beans are loaded with antioxidants that protect the cells from damages that can result in cancer, arthritis, heart disease, immune system problems, Alzheimer's and dementia.

Butternut Squash Soup

1 medium butternut squash
1 large onion – chopped
1 stalk of celery– chopped
1 large apple – peeled and sliced
½ t salt or to taste
Parsley leaves for garnish

1. Using vegetable peeler, peel butternut squash to the orange-color flesh. Cut of ends, cut in half and scoop out seeds. Slice into slices or cut squash into chunks.
2. In a large sauce pan, add 2 tablespoons water over medium heat until bubbly. Sauté onions until they are translucent. Add squash, celery and 4 cups of water cook until vegetables are soft. Add apple slices; season with salt to taste. Let cool.
3. Blend the soup in a food processor or blender until smooth (or chunky if you prefer) in several batches. Reheat gently over low heat. Stir frequently. Garnish with parsley leaves.

Nutritionally this winter squash offers many health benefits. Study shows that winter squash to be the number one source of alpha-carotene and beta-carotene. No other single food provides greater percentage of certain carotenoids than winter squash. Its antioxidant and anti-inflammatory compounds have shown this food to have clear potential in cancer prevention and cancer treatment such as in prostate, colon, breast and lung cancers.

Cool Pea Soup

1 c raw cashews - soak in 1 c water
2 c frozen peas or fresh garden peas
¼ onions – chopped or 1 t onion powder
1 t salt to taste
2 c water

1. Place all ingredients in blender. Blend it until very smooth and creamy. If double recipe, you can process in batches.
2. Refrigerate until ready to serve. Use it within a day or two.

This recipe takes only a few minutes to prepare. You can adjust the creaminess according to taste - use more cashews and less water for a thicker creamier consistency.

The Pea Soup is equally welcome as a hot soup. Just drop the peas in boiling water, let it boil for 2 minutes. Let cool. Process it in the blender until smooth. Reheat.

Green peas are one of the most nutritious leguminous vegetables, rich in protein, fiber, phytonutrients and antioxidants which help to protect from lung and oral cavity cancers. Fresh peas are excellent source of folic acid and B-complex vitamins required for DNA synthesis inside the cell. Fresh peas are also rich in vitamin C, a powerful antioxidant that helps body scavenge harmful free radicals. Peas contain B-sitosterol which helps lower cholesterol levels. In addition, green peas contain vitamin K important in building bone mass and protecting neuronal damage in the brain.

Avocado and Apple Soup

1 ripe avocado
1 unpeeled apple – cut
1 t lemon juice
2 c water
½ t salt to taste

Put all ingredients in a blender. Process it until smooth. If too thick, add more water to desired consistency. Serve chilled.

I was puzzled as what to serve when one of my family members had a tooth extraction and needed a liquid diet for a couple of days. That's how this recipe came about. The Avocado-Apple Soup also freezes well and can be served as a frozen dessert.

This enzyme - rich soup is another way to serve avocados. This fruit is rich in vitamins A, C, E, K, B6, folate, copper, potassium, calcium and magnesium. It is also a good source of fiber. A medium avocado contains around 30 grams of fat, but about 20 grams are mono-unsaturated fats (oleic acid) which are beneficial for health. The oleic acid in avocados may prevent certain types of cancer like prostate cancer. The fruit also have anti-inflammatory and antioxidant properties that prevent healthy cells from turning malignant, and also cause death of cancer cells.

Eating avocados can help lower cholesterol levels and reduce triglyceride levels in blood. Because avocado is rich in potassium and folate which helps to lower the risk of heart diseases and stroke.

SALADS

Pickled Vegetable Salad
Kale Kraut Salad
Kale, Broccoli, and Carrot Salad with Almond Dressing
Barley and Vegetable Salad
Potato Salad
Carrot and Daikon Salad
Carrot - Sunflower Seeds with Avocado Cream Dressing
Kidney Bean Avocado Salad
Noodle Salad with Almond Butter Sauce
Red Kidney Bean Salad with Yogurt Dressing
Quinoa and Black Bean Salad
Shari's Rainbow Salad
Lentils and Arugula Salad
Rainbow Bell Peppers
Simple Zucchini Salad

Fresh raw vegetables and raw fruits contain valuable enzymes which are destroyed by cooking. Remember, enzymes are living elements, the "life" in your food. Include more raw and living foods every day as toppings for soups, in salads, in sandwiches and wraps. You can grow sprouts in your own kitchen.

Salads made with beans, pasta and noodles or grains can be considered as main dishes. When combined with sufficient raw vegetables they are hearty and substantial as a one dish meal.

Pickled Vegetable Salad

1 c Napa cabbage or regular cabbage – sliced
1 Persian cucumber – sliced
½ c celery – diced
¼ c red radishes – sliced
¼ c red onion – chopped
1 t salt or to taste

1. Put all ingredients in a large bowl. Using gloved-hand to gently massage the vegetables until liquid begins to come out.
2. Place a plate on top of vegetables inside the bowl, and put weights on top of plate to squeeze out the liquid for about one-hour.
3. Drain the liquid (save for other uses) before serving.

This is a very simple salad that is chock full of enzymes and fiber. Cabbage contains active components that block certain cancers due to its antioxidants, anti-inflammatory activities, and glucosinolates. Glucosinolates are sulfur containing substances in green cabbage with exceptional cancer preventive properties for bladder, colon, and prostate cancer. Radishes contribute a good supply of vitamin C.

Kale Kraut Salad

1 bunch organic kale (dinosaur "lacinato" flat or curly leaves)
1 T extra virgin olive oil*
2–3 t fresh lemon juice to desire tartness
¼ – ½ t salt to taste
¼ t cayenne powder or to taste, optional

1. Remove kale's tough center ribs. Save for cooking or juicing.
2. Finely chop kale leaves and place in a large bowl.
3. Add seasonings.
4. Using gloved-hand massage kale with seasonings combined.
5. Transfer to serving platter; and surround with avocados and tomatoes, if desire.
   *Oil-less version (omit the olive oil) – add one avocado.

The Kale Kruat Salad makes a pleasant change from the common lettuce-type salad. I prefer the flat leaves known as dinosaur or black, lacinato or Tuscan. They have a nutty taste. The curly leaves which are bright green taste more tart and spicier.

Kale is especially rich in calcium, iron, magnesium and trace minerals, vitamins A, C, E, K, and the B vitamins. Instead of kale, you can use other green vegetables as collards, chard or other greens. The greens also provide glucosinolates which help fight cancer. The kale, collards, broccoli, and other greens have as much calcium as cow's milk. Since these are organic calcium from raw vegetables, unlike the inorganic calcium in pasteurized cow's milk, they are much easier for the body to absorb and assimilate.

Kale, Broccoli, and Carrot Salad with Almond Dressing

5 cups organic kale – chopped (remove center ribs for other uses)
1 c organic broccoli florets
½ organic carrot – shredded

Dressing:
1 c cooked or canned beans (pinto, white or navy beans)
¼ cup raw almond butter
½ cup water
1 T lemon juice
2 cloves garlic – chopped
1 T fresh ginger – grated
4 pitted dates
1 T miso paste
1 t salt

1. In a large bowl combine kale, broccoli and shredded carrots
2. Blend all dressing ingredients in a blender until creamy. Add a little water if too thick
3. Wearing gloves pour half of the dressing over the kale.
   Massage well into the vegetables. Save remainder dressing in a jar for dips or over cooked vegetables, potatoes, rice or pasta.

This salad is full of anti-cancer benefits. The spotted pinto beans are rich in antioxidants and fiber. Just one cup of pinto beans provides 73 percent of our daily recommended need for folate, which has been shown to reduce the risk of heart disease and breast cancer. Raw almond butter is an excellent source of selenium, a powerful antioxidant. Almonds contain protein, fiber, vitamin E, calcium and magnesium. Dates are rich in fiber, B-vitamins; it has more potassium than bananas, and more selenium than spinach. Kale, broccoli and carrots contain powerful anti-cancer phytochemicals.

Barley and Vegetable Salad

4 c cooked whole barley
6 oz. organic fresh spinach – chopped
1-2 green onions or scallions - chopped
1 T grated lemon zest
1 cucumber – thinly sliced
1 large or 2 medium tomatoes – chopped
1 T apple cider vinegar
2 sun-dried tomatoes (no oil), rehydrated; then finely chopped
1 garlic clove – finely chopped
2 T Bragg Liquid Aminos
Salt to taste

1. In a large bowl, toss together the first 6 ingredients (barley, spinach, green onions, lemon zest, cucumbers and tomatoes).
2. In a smaller bowl whisk together the apple cider vinegar, sun-dried tomatoes, garlic, liquid aminos.
3. Pour the dressing over the barley and vegetables. Toss together and season with salt to taste. May garnish with additional sprinkles of lemon zest if desire.

Whole grain barley provides a good source of protein, complex carbohydrate, some calcium and vitamin E. The fiber in barley helps to speed the passages of carcinogens; also binds lipids and other toxins and wastes through the digestive tract to be eliminated via the colon.

Spinach furnishes many important vitamins, minerals, antioxidants and cancer fighting phytonutrients. Tomatoes are one of the best dietary sources of lycopene. Research has shown that lycopene can stop cancer cell growth.

Potato Salad

2 lbs. organic potatoes (7–8 medium size)
1 organic red bell pepper – diced
3 organic celery stalks – diced
1 organic green apple – diced
½ small red onion – sliced
1 green onion – sliced, optional
1 c soy yogurt (see recipe under Yogurt)
Salt and onion powder to taste

1. Cook potatoes. Peel and dice.
2. In a large bowl, mix remaining ingredients.
3. Season with salt and onion powder to taste.

This Potato Salad does not contain oil or fat. It is best served immediately, as the yogurt tends to disappear into the potatoes if kept more than one or two days.

Red bell peppers contain powerful antioxidants which can help prevent several cancers: stomach, colon, breast, prostate and lung. A serving of red bell peppers provides almost 300 percent of the daily vitamin C intake. It is also rich in vitamin B6 and magnesium that helps to decrease blood pressure and anxiety.

Carrot – Sunflower Seeds with Avocado Cream Dressing

5 organic carrots
1 T apple cider vinegar
2 T cilantro or parsley – chopped

Seasoned sunflower seeds:
½ c raw sunflower (pumpkin seeds) – soak 10 minutes, drain
¼ t salt
Pinch of cayenne powder, optional

Dressing:
2 avocados
1 T lemon juice
1– 2 t white miso paste
½ t onion powder
2–4 T water, as needed

1. In a food processor, using the slicing/shredding disk grate the carrots. Toss together in a large bowl shredded carrots, apple cider vinegar and cilantro/parsley.
2. In a small bowl, mix soaked and drained sunflower seeds with salt and cayenne, if using.
3. Use half of the seasoned seeds and combine with the carrot mixture. Reserve the remaining seeds as garnish.
4. Blend avocados, lemon juice, white miso paste, onion powder and water in a blender until smooth. May add more water if needed. Place half of the avocado cream into the carrot mixture. Combine well.
5. Divide into 4 equal portions on salad plates. Place a dollop of the avocado cream on top of the carrot mixture. Sprinkle with remaining seeds and garnish with cilantro or parsley leaves.

Carrots contain many disease-fighting properties and anti-cancer activity. Carrots help in maintaining healthy epithelial tissues surrounding the internal organs. These epithelial tissues are susceptible to cancerous growth. Both pumpkin seeds and sunflower seeds contain iron, zinc, magnesium, potassium and calcium; the B vitamins and vitamin E. Avocado lowers cholesterol, controls blood pressure and smooth skin. Because the ingredients in this dish are raw, all heat sensitive vitamins, and live enzymes remain viable.

Kidney Bean Avocado Salad

4 c cooked or canned kidney beans, drained
2 tomatoes – chopped
1 green bell pepper – chopped
2 green onions – chopped
1 large avocado
1 T lemon juice
½ t salt or to taste
½ t crushed red chili peppers

Mix all ingredients in a large bowl. Chill and serve.

Kidney beans contain cancer fighting selenium; immune boosting zinc; and antioxidant rich vitamin E. The red kidney beans are exceptionally rich in flavonoids that have anti-aging properties. In fact, red kidney beans contain more flavonoids than blueberries. In addition, kidney beans are full of folates and fiber - both are protective against cancer, heart disease and stroke. Of course tomatoes are rich in lycopene, powerful antioxidant that help the body resist cancer and its progression.

Noodle Salad with Almond Butter Sauce

1 lb. linguini noodles (wide-flat ones)
3–4 cups thinly sliced vegetables (arugula, kale, red cabbage, Napa cabbage, spinach, collards, any leafy vegetables or lettuce greens)
1 t Balsamic vinegar, optional
1 cucumber – slice to match sticks
1 red bell pepper – chopped
1 green onions – chopped
½ c cilantro – chopped
½ c almond slices, optional for garnish

Sauce:
3 dates soaked in 1 ¼ c water
½ cup creamy almond butter
3–4 T Bragg Liquid Aminos to taste
1 T lemon juice or1 T apple cider vinegar to taste
1 clove garlic – chopped
1 thumb-size fresh ginger – chopped
1 red or green chili pepper, optional

1. Cook linguini noodles according to directions on the package. While cooking the noodles, toss the greens with 1 t Balsamic vinegar and set aside.
2. In a large container, toss noodles, vinegar-seasoned vegetables, cucumber, bell pepper, onions and cilantro.
3. In a blender, blend the sauce ingredients until smooth. Add more water if prefer a thinner sauce.
4. Pour the sauce over the noodles and vegetables. Mix well.

This dish can be served as a one-dish meal. If you like cucumbers, you can use more. Let me tell you why:

The humble cucumber contains more health benefits than we realize. Its peel is a good source of dietary fiber that helps reduce constipation; and offers some protection against colon cancers by eliminating toxic compounds from the gut. Cucumber supplies potassium which is heart friendly by reducing blood pressure and heart rates. Cucumbers' antioxidants act as protective scavengers against damaging free radicals in cancer, aging and disease processes.

The Noodle Salad with Almond Butter Sauce is full of rainbow colored vegetables rich in the flavonoids that provide antioxidants and anti-cancer phytonutrients. The noodles with nutrient rich almond butter provide protein, fiber, calcium, magnesium, vitamin E and fiber.

Red Kidney Bean Salad with Yogurt Dressing

3 c cooked or canned red kidney beans with ¼ c liquid
1– 2 stalks of tender celery – chopped
1 Persian cucumber – chopped
2 T onions – chopped, optional
1/3 c soy yogurt (see recipe under Yogurt)
1 T lemon juice to taste
½ t salt or to taste

Toss all ingredients in a large bowl and serve.

I prefer to buy the dried beans and soak them overnight. Next day, drain the beans and place in a large pot with fresh water and cook until done. Save extra cooked beans in the freezer for soups.

All legumes and beans provide essential nutrients necessary for every cell in our body. Red kidney beans, in particular, contain the highest antioxidants important in sustaining good health. One cup of red beans provides half of your daily requirement of fiber, which keeps the digestive system healthy, prevents constipation, lowers cholesterol levels, and regulates blood sugar levels.

Quinoa and Black Bean Salad

1 c quinoa
½ red onion – chopped fine
1 c cooked corn
4 c cooked black beans or canned black beans, rinsed and drained
1 c cilantro – chopped fine
1 green onion – chopped fine
2 fresh tomatoes – chopped fine
2 T lemon juice
1 T apple cider vinegar
1 t garlic powder
1 t salt or to taste
1 avocado – chopped fine
Onion powder to taste, optional
1 cucumber – chopped fine, optional

1. Quinoa requires soaking and then thoroughly rinsed before cooking to wash off its naturally bitter coating (saponin). Put 1 cup quinoa in 2 cups water in a sauce pan. Bring to boil, reduce heat. Simmer for 15-18 minutes. Set aside. Yield 3 c cooked quinoa. Fluff with fork, set aside to cool.
2. In a large bowl, combine all remaining ingredients. Mix well.
3. Add cooked quinoa and toss together. Serve with lemon wedges if desire.

This recipe delivers a unique blend of sweet, tart and bland flavors that seems to be a hit with most taste buds. The ingredients in this recipe help lower the cholesterol, stabilize blood sugar, combat cancer and prevent constipation. Black beans provide an abundant supply of antioxidants and minerals.

Quinoa, an ancient grain, is packed with complete protein higher than other grains. It is also rich in calcium, magnesium, iron, phosphorus, and potassium. Quinoa can help lower cholesterol, blood pressure and the risk of heart disease.

Shari's Rainbow Salad

1 package (7oz.) arugula
1 c cooked kamut
1 c cooked or canned garbanzo beans
1 c corn
1 avocado – diced
1 yellow, orange or red bell pepper – diced
1 c cherry or grape tomatoes
1–2 fresh figs (mango or other fruit) – diced
1 small red onions – sliced
1 c tofu – cubed

1. Put all ingredients except tofu cubes in a large salad bowl. Toss gently.
2. Place tofu cubes on top. Chill and serve dressing of your choice on the side or just spray with Bragg Liquid Aminos.

Our daughter Shari enjoys cooking ever since a little girl. Guests always enjoy her salads. Here is a sample of one of her creations that even appeals to a toddler:

One day at lunch time, a friend with her 2½ year-old toddler came by for a visit while Shari was eating her salad. After offering her salad to the friend who had eaten already, the toddler blurted out, "Can I have some your salad?" "Sure, what would you like?"

"I want some beans, corn, tomatoes.....and I want some those, those green leaves."

"Those are arugula, you may not like them."

After chewing on the arugula momentarily, the little girl exclaimed, "I *love* them! I want more..!"

Arugula is a cruciferous vegetable associated with reduced risk of cancer. Its valuable antioxidants help to protect the body from skin cancer, lung cancer, and oral cancer. Arugula is rich in sulforaphane which has excellent chemo-protective effects and fights carcinogens.

Some may not have tasted kamut (pronounce "kah - moot.") It is a specialty whole grain; heirloom wheat originally came from Egypt. Kamut has a naturally sweet, buttery flavor. Soak the grains first and then cook them. Kamut is easier to digest and can be tolerated by people who are allergic or sensitive to wheat. It is rich in protein, approximately 30 percent more than wheat. Kamut provides dietary fiber that lowers risk of heart disease, stroke, high cholesterol, high blood pressure, diabetes, colon cancer, and constipation. It has anti-aging properties due to its high content of selenium and zinc.

Figs are a good source of potassium and fiber. Study with postmenopausal women consuming the most fruit fiber showed a 34 percent reduction in breast cancer. Among those who had used hormone replacement, it was noted that those consuming the most fiber, especially cereal fiber (kamut), had a 50 percent reduction in their risk of breast cancer compared to those consuming the least.

Lentils and Arugula Salad

2 c lentils – cleaned and rinsed
3 ¾ c water
1 t sage powder
1 t rosemary powder
1 T onion powder
1 t salt or to taste
1 package (7oz.) arugula
2 tomatoes – chopped
1 avocado – diced
2 T red onions – chopped, optional
Raw shelled hemp seeds, optional

1. Put lentils and water in a sauce pan and bring to boil. Add sage, rosemary and onion powder. Simmer on low until lentils are tender but firm ~15 minutes.
2. Add salt and continue simmer until desired tenderness and most liquids are absorbed ~10 minutes with lid off. Drain and save broth for other uses.
3. Serve lentils over arugula greens on individual plates. Top with tomatoes, avocados, red onions and sprinkle raw shelled hemp seeds.

Two cups of lentils will yield approximately 5 cups of cooked lentils. The cooked lentils can be served either hot or cold over the arugula greens.

For a quick one-dish meal, just buy a box of Trader Joe's "Steamed Lentils Ready to Eat Warm or Cold" in the refrigerated section. Mix lentils with a jar of bruschetta (no sugar). Serve with any greens you have.

Arugula is rich in antioxidants which protects the body from cancers. It also provides vitamin K known to promote bone health and brain function.

Lentils contain one of the highest amounts of protein among plants up to 35 percent which is comparable to meat, poultry, fish, and dairy products. Lentils also provide phytochemicals that can control cancer growth.

Rainbow Bell Peppers

1 red, 1 green and 1 yellow or purple bell peppers
1 small red onion
1 cucumber
1 zucchini
1 fresh fruit (apple, mango, persimmon, peach)
1 tomato
1 avocado
1 chili or jalapeno pepper
1 T olive oil
2 t lemon juice to taste
½ t salt or to taste
Cilantro for garnish

1. Dice all ingredients to desired bite size in a large bowl.
2. Add seasonings and garnish. Chill and serve.

This salad offers a high content of phytochemicals with an abundance of cancer fighting nutrients.

Simple Zucchini Salad

1 zucchini – diced
½ t onion powder
Salt to taste
Sprays of Bragg Liquid Aminos to taste
Cayenne powder, optional

Toss all ingredients together. Chill and serve.

One cup of zucchini provides 10 percent of our daily requirement for fiber. The fiber help prevent carcinogenic toxins in the colon. Zucchini also contain powerful antioxidants that fight oxidative stress that can lead to cancer. The summer squash contains anti-inflammatory agents that can deter the development of many hyper-inflammatory disorders. In addition, zucchini can help lower cholesterol, lower blood pressure, and promote healthy skin.

SALAD DRESSINGS

Soy Yogurt Dressing
Bragg Liquid Aminos and Sesame Dressing
White Bean and Veggie Dressing
All Purpose Salad Dressing
Tofu Salad Dressing
Creamy Cucumber Dressing
Creamy Avocado – Cucumber Dressing
Persimmon Dressing

Soy Yogurt Dressing

One pint jar homemade soy yogurt (see recipe under Yogurt)
2–3 T Ketchup*
½ small red or sweet onions – chopped
1 t onion powder, optional
Salt to taste

1. Put ketchup, chopped onions, onion powder and salt into a jar of homemade yogurt.
2. Mix well and refrigerate.

The Soy Yogurt Dressing is a basic creamy dressing that goes well with lettuce type greens, potato salad, beans and grain- type salads. If you prefer a stronger flavor, add some minced garlic, chili peppers or ginger. These pungent spices support the immune system, combat cancer, reduce inflammation, and perk up appetite.

*Organic Ville Organic Ketchup with agave nectar.

Bragg Liquid Aminos and Sesame Dressing

½ c liquid aminos
½ t pure sesame oil

Mix well in a glass jar with lid.

This dressing can be used over rice, noodles, tofu, salads or any dish for an Asian twist. We often put this dressing in a dropper bottle with a screw-lid that I tuck in my purse whenever we go out to eat or travel on the road. Most commercial salad dressings contain refined oil, sugar, corn syrup, and chemical additives.

White Bean and Veggie Dressing

1 15-oz. can white beans or 1 ½ cups of cooked white beans
2– 3 T lemon juice or to taste
1 t olive oil, optional
1 t salt
½ c parsley – chopped
¼ of small onion – chopped

1. Drain canned beans or cooked dried beans.
2. In a blender, puree beans, lemon juice, olive oil if using and salt until smooth. Add a little water if needed for smoothness.
3. Add chopped parsley and onions. Puree until well blended.

Beans have protein, fiber and rich in minerals. White kidney beans or cannellini beans contain the highest amount of iron among beans. Kidney beans (red or white) are also rich in vitamin K an important vitamin for bones. The antioxidants in white beans can keep normal cells from turning cancerous.

Parsley has several anticancer activities: blocking receptor sites for certain cancer promotion; resisting cancer formation; and stimulating the beneficial enzymes to detoxify carcinogens. Onions also have similar benefits as parsley which can inhibit growth of cancer cells and eliminate carcinogens.

All Purpose Salad Dressing

½ cup water
2 dates soaked in 2 T water
2 T lemon juice or to taste
2 T Dijon mustard, optional
2 T Miso
2 T nutritional yeast

Blend all ingredients in a blender until smooth.

Miso provides beneficial bacteria and enzymes for digestion. It strengthens the immune system and combats viral infection.

Mustard seed contain phytonutrients called – isothiocyanates which have anti-cancer effect. Isothiocyanates has been shown to inhibit growth of existing cancer cells and protect against the formation of new cancer cells.

Tofu Salad Dressing

1 box soft tofu (~19 oz.)
2 T lemon juice or to taste
3 T apple cider vinegar
1 T agave nectar
1 t Dijon mustard – optional
2 T red onions – finely chopped
2 t lemon zest
1 t salt or to taste
1 t onion powder
Pinch of dill weed, optional

1. Blend in blender tofu, lemon juice, apple cider vinegar, agave, Dijon mustard, if using until smooth. Add water if too thick one tablespoon at a time. Transfer to a bowl.
2. Stir in onions, lemon zest, salt, onion powder and dill weed, if using. Store it in glass jar in refrigerator. Yield: 3 cups.

Tofu supplies protein, calcium, vitamins, minerals, protecting against heart disease and cancer. Tofu is rich in isoflavones which can reduce risk of osteoporosis, breast, and prostate cancers.

Creamy Cucumber Dressing

1 c raw sunflower seeds
1 cucumber with skin, coarsely chopped
½ c lemon juice
1 t onion powder
1 c water
1 t maple syrup or agave nectar
Pinch of rosemary powder

Blend all ingredients in blender until creamy.

Raw sunflower seeds are a good source of selenium. Selenium has been shown to induce DNA repair and synthesis in damaged cells, and also inhibit the proliferation of cancer cells. Sunflower seeds contain a rich supply of vitamin E which has been shown to reduce the risk of colon cancer, bladder cancer, and prostate cancer.

Cucumbers provide fiber which is beneficial for colon health. Cucumbers also contain cancer-fighting antioxidants, and a rich source of minerals.

Creamy Avocado – Cucumber Dressing

1 whole cucumber – chopped with skin on
¼ cup water
1 avocado
1 T fresh lemon juice
1 t salt or to taste
1 t onion powder
1 t agave nectar, optional

1. Put cucumber and water in blender. Blend until smooth.
2. Add remaining ingredients, blend until creamy.

Persimmon Dressing

2 ripe persimmons
Juice of 1 orange, ~1/3 c
1 – 2 t lemon juice or to taste
¼ t turmeric
½ t onion powder
1/8 t salt or to taste
Dehydrated minced onions, optional

1. Place ingredients in blender and blend until smooth.
2. Sprinkle dehydrated minced onions on top. Serve over fruit or vegetable salad.

You can use fresh mangoes or fresh peaches instead of persimmons. This oriental fruit contain an anti-tumor compound called betulinic acid. Fresh persimmons contain many antioxidants that function as scavengers against free radicals that play a role in cancer, aging and various disease processes.

VEGETABLES

Steamed Asparagus Spears
Baked Zucchini with Onions
Roasted Vegetable Medley
Baked Onions
Caramelized Onions
Roasted Potatoes
Sauté Yucca Root with Onions and Garlic
Sautéed Button Mushrooms
Basil and Shiitake Mushrooms
Healthy Kimchi
Bowtie Kelp and Cilantro
Pickled Turnip Greens
Garlic Roasted Brussels Sprouts

Steamed Asparagus Spears

1 package frozen asparagus spears
2 t onion powder
1 t salt to taste
2 sprays of Bragg Liquid Aminos
2 drops of pure sesame seed oil, optional

1. In a large skillet, place frozen asparagus spears with 4 T water. Cover and cook over low-medium heat.
2. While steaming, add onion powder and salt. Continue cooking till tender. Spray liquid aminos to taste.
3. Remove from heat. Add one or two drops of sesame seed oil.

History tells us that the King of France (Louis XIV) enjoyed asparagus so much that he had special green houses built so he could enjoy asparagus year-round. Asparagus contains a protein called histones which is believed to control cell growth that may be beneficial for cancer. Asparagus also contains glutathione, a powerful antioxidant and a detoxifying compound. Glutathione breaks down carcinogens in the body, and it also boosts immune cells. According to the National Cancer Institute's "The Glutathione Report," asparagus is the highest tested food containing this powerful antioxidant. Other vegetables (avocados, kale, Brussels sprouts) also contain glutathione.

Baked Zucchini with Onions

2 zucchini – sliced horizontally
1 onion – sliced
1 t dried sage, optional
½ t salt or to taste
Bragg Liquid Aminos

1. In a large bowl toss the zucchini and onion slices with the seasonings.
2. Put in a baking dish. Spray vegetables with the liquid aminos.
3. Cover and bake at 400°F for 15 minutes. Remove cover and continue baking for 15 minutes or until tender.

Italians used zucchini as a cure-all. Its antioxidants can protect our cells against oxidative damage.

Roasted Vegetable Medley

8-10 shiitake mushrooms – quartered and marinate in:
2 T liquid aminos
¼ – ½ c water
1 t onion powder
2 Japanese eggplant – slice in rounds
2 carrots – cut in baby-carrot-size sticks
1 small red or yellow or white onion – sliced
Bragg Liquid Aminos

Vegetable coating:
1 T arrowroot powder or cornstarch
1 t salt
1 chili pepper – minced
1 t fresh ginger- minced
3 cloves garlic – minced
1 t garlic powder

1. Marinate mushrooms. Set aside.
2. In a large bowl, put arrowroot powder, salt, chili pepper, ginger, garlic and garlic powder. Add eggplant slices, carrots and onions. Mix and coat the vegetables well.
3. Place in a baking pan and spray with squirts of liquid aminos over the vegetables.
4. Put the marinated mushrooms on top of vegetables. Pour ~1/4 c water at bottom of baking pan. Cover with lid.
5. Bake at 400°F for 45 minutes or until vegetables and mushrooms are tender.

You can use other vegetables in this recipe. Most roasting or baking can be done without oil. Heated fats can generate carcinogens. Instead, I use arrowroot powder or cornstarch to coat the vegetables.

Eggplant provides important phytonutrients. One phytonutrient, anthocyanin, is found on the eggplant skin is called nasunin. This antioxidant has been shown to protect the brain cells in animal studies. Eggplant contains another compound called chlorogenic acid which is one of the most potent free radical scavengers that provides anti-cancer and antimicrobial benefits.

Mushrooms contain cancer-fighting and immune-boosting compounds to fight against cancer and the common cold.

Baked Onions

1 red onion and 1 yellow sweet onion – sliced
2 t Balsamic vinegar in 1 T water
Bragg Liquid Aminos

1. Place onion slices in a baking dish with cover.
2. Pour Balsamic vinegar-water over onions slices.
3. Spray with liquid aminos over the onions.
4. Cover and bake at 250° F for 2–3 hours until done.

Onions are rich in flavonoids that are protective against cancers. Flavonoids in onion tend to be more concentrated in the outer layers of the flesh. To maximize your health benefits, peel off as little of the fleshy edible portion as possible when removing the onion's outermost paper-layer. A red onion can lose about 20 percent of its quercetin (a flavonoid) and almost 75 percent of its anthocyanins (another flavonoid) if it is over peeled.

Caramelized Onions

3 medium size onions – thinly sliced
¼ t salt or to taste

1. In a dry skillet, sauté onions over medium heat. Add salt.
2. Cook onions until they begin to caramelize to golden-brown. Approximately 10 to 15 minutes. Stir often.

The Caramelized Onions taste sweet as they become caramelized. This recipe makes a delicious side dish with pasta, potatoes, rice, vegetables, entrees, and in sandwiches.

Just by eating several servings of onion each week is sufficient to statistically lower one's risk of certain cancers such as colorectal, laryngeal, and ovarian cancer. To combat oral and esophageal cancer, one needs to consume approximately ½ cup of onions per day.

Roasted Potatoes

6-8 Organic Russet Potatoes – cut into wedges, leave the skins on

Coating:
1 T arrowroot powder or cornstarch
1 T onion powder
1 t salt
4 cloves garlic – minced
¼ t rosemary powder, optional

1. Place arrowroot powder, onion powder, salt, garlic and rosemary powder in a large bowl.
2. Toss potato wedges with the coating until well mixed.
3. Place in baking pan. Squirt sprays of liquid aminos over the potatoes.
4. Bake @400°F with cover on for ~45 minutes. Take off cover, continue baking 5 - 10 minutes or until done.

Organic potatoes taste delicious. When it is roasted with the skin and without oil potato actually is a good food. Although potatoes are high in the glycemic index (GI) which can raise blood sugar quickly; but when eaten with the skins along with other whole foods at the same meal, the GI drops. Potatoes are fat free, rich in fiber, iron, B vitamins, vitamin C, potassium and magnesium. You can also roast some onions with the potatoes.

Sauté Yucca Root with Onions and Garlic

1 ~10 inch yucca root – peel with sharp knife or vegetable peeler
1 small onion – diced
5-8 cloves garlic – diced
Salt to taste
½ t cumin to taste
Cilantro – chopped for garnish

1. Cut peeled yucca root into wedges. Cover with water. Season it with salt. Bring to boil, simmer until tender ~15 – 20 minutes. Do not overcook. Take out of water and save cooking broth. Remove and discard the hard veins in center of yucca root. Dice yucca to bite size.
2. In a skillet, sauté onions and garlic in little cooking broth. Add diced yucca root and cumin to taste. Add more cooking broth as needed. Stir in cilantro. Enjoy while warm.

Yucca root makes a nice alternative to potatoes. Its outer skin is brown, inside is white. It provides many health benefits. Yucca's antioxidants can protect the body from damage caused by oxidation that can lead to cancer and cardiovascular diseases. Yucca roots can stop the buildup of oxygen free radicals, and prevent blood vessel damages. Consumption of this humble root helps to control blood sugar, blood pressure, and cholesterol levels. The root also contains anti-inflammatory properties that can aid in reducing the swelling and pain of arthritis, bursitis, and gout.

Sautéed Button Mushrooms

1 10 oz. package whole button mushrooms (~20) – quartered
cloves garlic – sliced
3 T parsley – chopped
½ t salt
Bragg Liquid Aminos

1. Put ¼ cup water in skillet over medium heat.
2. Add garlic and cook until transparent, about 1 minute.
3. Add mushrooms and cook on low heat with lid on for 10 minutes without stirring.
4. Add half of parsley, salt and liquid aminos to taste. Stir briefly.
5. Garnish with remaining parsley.

All ingredients in this recipe contain healing compounds. White button mushrooms contain an important cancer-fighting substance – conjugated linolenic acid (CLA) which reduces risk posed by high estrogen levels implicated in breast cancer. Studies showed that white mushrooms showed more promise for reducing cancer risk from high estrogen than other vegetables tested. Button mushrooms also reduce risk against prostate cancer.

Garlic not only decreases the risk of stomach, colon cancers, breast, esophageal cancers, but also reduces the LDL (bad) cholesterol, raises HDL (good) cholesterol, and lowers triglycerides and blood pressure.

Parsley provides carotenoids with anti-cancer and anti-inflammatory properties. Parsley is rich with chlorophyll, an excellent blood builder and purifier. Parsley is high in both vitamin C and iron which makes iron absorption more effective.

Basil and Shiitake Mushrooms

10–12 shiitake mushrooms – cut into quarters
3 garlic cloves – sliced
3" fresh ginger – sliced
3 c fresh basil leaves
1 stalk green onions – sliced
Salt to taste
1 t arrowroot powder
1 t Bragg Liquid Aminos
1/3 c water

1. Place 2 T water in the skillet over medium heat, sauté mushrooms, garlic and ginger for 5 minutes or until mushrooms are soft. Add basil leaves, green onions until wilted and season with salt to taste.
2. Mix arrowroot powder, liquid aminos and water in a small bowl. Pour over the mushrooms and greens, stir briefly until bubbly.

The Basil and Shiitake Mushrooms is a favorite in Chinese restaurants. Although in the restaurants most dishes are cooked with lots of oil and refined sugar.

Shiitake mushrooms contain several compounds with health benefits. A compound called lentinan is believed to stop or slow tumor growth. Another component – 1, 3 beta glucan can reduce tumor activity and lessen the side effects of cancer treatment. Shiitake mushrooms also contain eritadenine which can lower cholesterol levels.

Basil is considered as the king of herbs revered as "holy herb" in many traditions. Basil contains exceptionally high levels of antioxidants that protect from lung and oral cavity cancers. Basil has anti-inflammatory properties, protects the heart, controls blood pressure and a blood purifier.

Healthy Kimchi

1 large Napa cabbage – sliced
1 head green cabbage – sliced
1 ~10" daikon – shredded
1 carrot – shredded
2 green onions – chopped
2 Persian cucumbers – sliced, optional
6-7 cloves garlic - chopped fine
1 ginger (thumb size) – chopped fine
6 red chili peppers – chopped fine, optional
¼ cup lemon juice
1 T agave nectar
1/8 t cayenne powder, optional
3–4 T coarse salt, raw unprocessed

1. If you have a food processor, use the slicing disk to slice the Napa cabbage (the firm part) and the head cabbage. Otherwise just slice by hand to desired size.
2. Using shredding blade shred the daikon and carrot in the food processor. Place all ingredients in a very large bowl.
3. Using gloved-hand to massage the vegetables until well mixed. Place in glass jars and refrigerate.

This recipe yields approximately 6 pint-size jars of Kimchi. If it tastes too spicy, reduce the chili peppers or omit it altogether. This dish seems to perk up a waning appetite.

Most store-bought Kimchi contains sugar, MSG, additives, and refined salt. Regular table salt is processed. and contains anti-caking agents, dextrose (sugar), and chemical additives. The unprocessed salt contains over 60 naturally occurring trace minerals which are essential for good health. Unless a person is salt sensitive, the unrefined/unprocessed salt is safe to use; in fact they contribute the needed trace minerals often lacking in a diet of mostly refined foods.

Napa cabbage contains isothiocyanates which may lower the risk of lung cancer. Its high vitamin content also strengthens the immune system and reduces inflammatory processes. There is more calcium in Napa cabbage than other variety. Napa cabbage provides both soluble and insoluble fiber which can reduce the incidence of diverticular disease, high blood pressure, certain cancers and stroke. In addition, Napa cabbage provides vitamin K, important in bone health.

A person eats the green cabbage just once a week can reduce the risk of colon cancer by 60 percent. Cabbage is also a good detoxifier for the blood and removes toxins. Cabbage contains iodine which aids in proper functioning of the brain, nervous system, and the endocrine glands.

Daikon is also known as Oriental or Chinese radish. Daikon contains antioxidants that fight free radical damage. Research has shown that daikon juice helps prevent the formation of carcinogens and help the liver process toxins. Its high vitamin C content provides immune system support. The daikon leaves are an excellent source of calcium. Raw daikon juice can help dissolve mucus and phlegm.

I use lemon juice in many recipes, not only for its taste, but also because lemons contribute to the alkalinity balance in our body. We think of citrus fruits for their vitamin C, but there are many anti-cancer compounds in citrus fruits. These nutrients can help slow and block growth of cancer cells.

Bowtie Kelp and Cilantro

4 cups of bowtie kelp (~1.5 pounds)
½ cup warm water
1 T unrefined sugar
1 T Bragg Liquid Aminos
4 cloves garlic – minced
1 chili pepper – minced
½ c cilantro – chopped

1. Put all ingredients except cilantro in a sauce pan over medium heat until boil. Continue to simmer on low heat until kelp is tender, approximately 40 minutes. Add more water as needed.
2. Garnish with cilantro and serve.

This simple dish can be served either hot or cold. Seaweed combines well with vegetables. It also adds texture and flavor to tofu, soy, and gluten dishes. Seaweed is found in most Asian stores in the dehydrated form or fresh in the refrigerated section.

Seaweed or sea vegetables are rich in minerals including calcium, magnesium, iron, iodine, sodium and potassium. It also contains significant amounts of vitamins A, C, E, K; beta carotene, folate and B-vitamins. Cilantro provides flavor, texture, color and aids in digestion and a powerful detoxifier.

Pickled Turnip Greens

1 bunch organic turnip greens (stems and leaves) – chopped
1 t salt or to taste

1. Place chopped turnip greens in a large bowl. Add salt to taste.
2. Mix well and place in glass jars. Keep refrigerated.

Turnip greens is one the most nutritious vegetables even more nutritious than the roots. They provide antioxidants (vitamin E, vitamin C and beta-carotene) that can wipe out destructive free radicals. These antioxidants can fight against heart disease, lung disease, cancer and arthritis. One cup of cooked turnip greens provides 197 mg calcium, top other greens. When eaten raw, nearly one hundred percent of the calcium is absorbed.

Garlic Roasted Brussels Sprouts

1 package (12 oz.) Brussels sprouts (~12–15)
5 garlic cloves – chopped fine
1 T Balsamic vinegar
2 T Bragg Liquid Aminos
1 T arrowroot powder
2 t lemon zest
¼ t rosemary – chopped
¼ cup water

1. Cut Brussels sprouts into halves.
2. In a large bowl combine the remaining ingredients.
3. Toss Brussels sprouts with seasonings. Transfer to a baking pan with lid.
4. Bake at 400°F with lid on for 25 minutes. Uncover, continue baking for 10-15 minutes until vegetables are tender. Stir once to prevent burning.

Brussels sprouts are small leafy green buds resemble miniature cabbages. They are rich in protein, fiber, vitamins, minerals, and antioxidants. The phytochemicals in the Brussels sprouts offer protection from prostate, colon, endometrial, lung, and oral cavity cancers. These miniature cabbages are an excellent source of vitamin C, A and E which help protect the body by trapping harmful free radicals thereby protect us from cardiovascular diseases and age-related macular degeneration. Brussels sprouts contain an excellent source of vitamin K which strengthens bones; and help limiting neuronal damage in the brain that can prevent the onset of Alzheimer's disease.

SANDWICHES

Edamame Sandwich Spread
Black Bean Veggie Burger
Oat-Tofu-Nut Burgers
Cashew Nut Spread
Chickpeas and Cucumber Salad in Pita Pockets

Edamame Sandwich Spread

1 package shelled or in pods frozen Edamame soybeans
½ c raw walnuts
½ c cilantro – roughly chopped (leaves and stems)
1 green onion or ¼ small red or sweet onion – chopped
1 t salt or to taste
4 T lemon juice
¼ – ½ c water to get a smooth consistency

1. Follow cooking instructions on Edamame soybeans. Put cooked shelled edamame, walnuts, cilantro, onions, and salt in food processor. Process until finely chopped.
2. With motor running, add lemon juice and enough water to make a smooth paste.
3. Use as a sandwich spread on bread, crackers, pocket bread or in wraps.
4. Top with lettuce, other greens, cucumber slices, tomatoes, avocados, and sprouts.

Edamame green soybeans are rich in plant protein, over 10 grams per ½ cup serving. They contain all the essential amino acids, high in omega-3 fatty acids, minerals, and fiber. The green soybeans contain protective phytoestrogens and no cholesterol.

Raw walnuts provide omega-3 fatty acids, lower cholesterol, and lift mood. Cilantro is a natural diuretic, aids in digestion and prevents nausea. Cilantro is a powerful metal detoxifier for mercury, lead, and cadmium. Both cilantro and onions contain anti-bacterial and anti-viral properties.

Black Bean Veggie Burger

3 c cooked black beans (or one 29-oz can, rinsed and drained)
2 c cooked brown rice
1 c bread crumbs (~2 slices toast and ground to crumbs)
1/3 c red onions – finely chopped
2 small chili pepper – finely chopped, optional
3 T organic ketchup (Organic Ville Ketchup with agave nectar)
1 T garlic (4–5 garlic cloves) – minced
½ c raw walnuts – finely chopped
1 c carrot pulp (from carrot juice) or shredded carrots
½ cup nutritional yeast
½ c flaxseeds – finely ground
1 t salt
½ t cayenne pepper
1/3 c raw sesame seeds
1 t Bill's Baste and Marinade, optional
~1/3 c water or more as needed

1. Preheat oven to 400°F. Lightly oil a non-sticky baking pan.
2. In a food processor, pulse all ingredients until combined but not pureed. Slowly add water as needed until the mixture feels sticky enough to hold together, but not too wet (process in batches if necessary).
3. Let chill few minutes or overnight. Shape into 10-12 patties and bake for 25-30 minutes. Gently flip the patties halfway through to finish baking the other side.

Instead of baking, the burgers can be pan "fried" in a non-stick skillet without oil on low-medium heat, approximately 10 minutes on each side.

There are so many variations to a veggie burger. From a nutritional angle, I like the black bean veggie burger the best. Black beans are among the superstars in fighting colon and breast cancer; stabilize blood sugar, and lower cholesterol. Brown rice contains B-vitamins, vitamin E, minerals and trace minerals.

Onions, chili peppers and garlic all lower the risks for several types of cancers, and boost immune system. Walnuts slow cancer growth and protect against heart disease. Lycopene from tomatoes helps in endometrial, lung, prostate, and stomach cancers.

Carrots are rich in cancer fighting antioxidants. Carrots are cleansing, and in detoxifying the liver and reduce toxicity of the blood. The carrots' molecules are closest to human hemoglobin molecules, making it beneficial in blood-building.

Flaxseed was cultivated in Babylon as early as 3000 B.C. In the 8th century, King Charlemagne believed so strongly in the health benefits of flaxseeds that he passed laws requiring his subjects to consume it. Research indicates that flax seeds may reduce risks of certain cancers, such as breast, prostate, and colon cancer.

Sesame seeds contain anti-cancer compounds, and are rich in magnesium which also has anti-cancer properties, especially beneficial against colorectal cancer.

Oat-Tofu-Nut Burgers

3 c rolled oats
2 c walnuts – chopped
2 ½ c cold water
1 box firm tofu – squeeze excess water
¼ cup nutritional yeast
2 T onion powder
2 T garlic powder
¾ c fresh parsley leaves –chopped (or 1/3 c dried parsley flakes)
5 T Bill's Chik'nish seasoning

1. In a large bowl combine oats, walnuts, and water. Set aside.
2. In a separate bowl mash tofu with fork and add remaining ingredients. Mix well.
3. Transfer seasoned-mashed tofu into the oat-nut mixture. Combine and mix well.
4. Form burger patties to desired size. Pan "fry" in a non-stick skillet on low-medium heat 5 minutes each side until golden brown. Serve on buns/pocket bread or as patties with gravy.

This recipe originally came from a friend who serves them in her restaurant. Her omnivore customers rave about these burgers. I have modified her recipe to a healthier version.

Whole oats have been widely touted for their health benefits including lower risk for cancer, heart diseases, and diabetes. Oats contain potent antioxidant properties; and have a good supply of proteins, vitamins, minerals, and fiber.

Walnuts rank second only to blackberries in terms of antioxidant content. Walnuts antioxidants help to protect us from chronic diseases as cardiovascular, neurological, cancer, and aging.

Tofu contains more protein than meat minus the cholesterol. It reduces bad cholesterol and risk of heart disease. Tofu contains isoflavones which help women to maintain balanced hormone levels.

Cashew Nut Spread

2 c raw cashew - soaked overnight and drained
2 T nutritional yeast
1 T lemon juice
1 t onion powder
2 t white miso paste, optional
1 t salt or to taste
1 t dried oregano or basil
1/2 c parsley – chopped
1 tomato – chopped fine

1. Process cashews in the food processor to a paste.
2. Add ~1/2c water, nutritional yeast, lemon juice, onion powder, miso and salt until smooth. Add water if needed.
3. Add herbs, parsley, and tomatoes. Use pause button to combine.

You can use the Cashew Nut Spread on bread, crackers, or as a dip for vegetables.

Chickpeas and Cucumber Salad in Pita Pockets

1 ½ c cooked/canned chickpeas (garbanzo beans) – drained
1 garlic clove – minced
2–3 T water
1 t lemon juice
¼ t salt to taste
½ c cucumber – diced
1 tomato – diced
½ green bell peppers – finely chopped, (include seeds if tender)
1 green onion – green and white parts chopped
1 t lemon juice
½ t olive oil, optional
¼ t salt to taste
2 whole wheat pita bread – cut in halves

1. Mash chickpeas and water with a fork leaving some whole. Add garlic, lemon juice, and salt.
2. In a separate bowel combine cucumbers, tomatoes, bell peppers, green onions, lemon juice, olive oil if using, and salt.
3. You can warm the pita bread in a toaster oven if desire.
4. Fill seasoned chickpeas and seasoned raw vegetables in pita pockets. Makes four half pockets.

To cook chickpeas, soak for 2-3 hours, drain. Use fresh water, cover 1 inch above the beans. After boiling, then simmer on low until tender, about 1 ½ hours. You can also use the canned chickpeas.

The stuffed pita pockets offer a complete meal. Chickpeas provide excellent supply of protein, fiber, vitamins, minerals and trace minerals. The inexpensive legumes are rich in tryptophan, an essential amino acid that is a precursor to serotonin that regulates both mood and sleep.

Bell peppers should be eaten raw as cooking destroys many of their nutritional compounds. Bell peppers are rich with antioxidants and anti-inflammatory compounds for cancer prevention. One cup of raw bell peppers contains nearly 200 percent of daily requirement for vitamin C. Green bell peppers contain zeaxanthin which keeps your eyes healthy.

Cucumbers contain antioxidants that protect our cells from free radical damages. Cucumbers are rich in potassium. This mineral is heart friendly that can help to regulate blood pressure.

ENTRÉE OR MAIN DISHES

Stuffed Shiitake Mushrooms
Mock Tofu Fish
Marinated Gluten and Vegetables with Cashew Gravy
Tofu Steaks with Tomatoes and Chestnuts
Marinated Tofu Cutlets with Asparagus Sauce
Baked Tofu with Veggies
Curried Potato – Vegetable Medley
"Soy Steak" Jerky
Baked Shiitake Mushrooms and Onions
Portobello Mushroom Steaks and Sweet Onions
Portobello Mushrooms with Tofu-Ginger Sauce
Rice and Bean Casserole
Curry Tofu with Coconut Milk and Rice
Mexi-Fritters with Corn Salsa
Tofu Sticks with Sweet and Sour Sauce
Red Bean and Mushroom Meat Loaf
Rice Wraps
Cabbage Rolls
Stuffed Eggplant
Soy Bean-curd Sticks
Singapore Mock Chicken
Soy Bean-curd Mock Duck
Taro Root "Drum Sticks"
Spaghetti with Edamame Sauce
Eggplant, Sundried Tomatoes, Spinach, Edamame with Fusilli Pasta
Whole Grain Penne with Eggplant, Tomatoes, and Olives
Garbanzo Sauce over Pasta Noodles
Bowtie Kelp with Soy Curls
Butternut Squash Shepherd's Pie
Twice Baked Potatoes with Sunflower Seeds and Herbs
Mexi-Potatoes with Baby Bella and Guacamole

Stuffed Shiitake Mushrooms

20 – 24 large shiitake mushrooms, stems removed for stuffing

Stuffing:
~1 c stems from shiitake mushrooms – chopped fine
1 garlic – minced
1/3 c onions – chopped fine
½ cup firm tofu, squeeze excess liquid; add dash of turmeric
½ t dried basil
½ t salt or to taste
1 c cooked spinach – chopped fine
2 slices whole wheat toast

Gravy:
1 c water
1 T arrowroot powder or cornstarch
1 T Bragg Liquid Aminos or soy sauce to taste

1. Select same size shiitake mushrooms. Gently twist off stems. Place whole mushrooms face up in a baking pan with lid.
2. Place a little water in skillet over medium heat. Sauté the chopped mushroom stems, garlic, onions, and crumbed tofu. Add seasonings, chopped spinach. Set aside to cool
3. Pulverize the toasted bread in food processor or Vita-mix. Add bread crumbs to the stuffing. Mix well.
4. Fill each mushroom with the stuffing. Pour a little water at the bottom of baking pan and cover with lid.
5. Bake @350°F for 15-20 minutes until mushrooms are tender.
6. Place the gravy ingredients in a small sauce pan, stir and cook over medium heat until thickened. Pour over the baked mushrooms just before serving. Serve warm.

Instead of shiitake mushrooms, you can use large button mushrooms. Reduced the baking time to 8-10 minutes and bake it without the lid. Instead of spinach, use cooked kale, collards, mustard greens, Swiss chard or other cooked greens. They all contain cancer-fighting antioxidants, minerals, and vitamins.

Shiitake mushrooms contain immune-supportive components known as polysaccharides that have been shown to reduce toxins, radiation exposures, stress, and immune-deficiency. Mushrooms also contain glyco-nutrients (essential sugars), similar to essential amino acids in protein foods.

Mock Tofu Fish

1 package oyster mushrooms
½ block of firm tofu, wrap in towel to remove moisture
½ t salt or to taste
1 T onion powder
2–3 T whole wheat flour
Bragg Liquid Aminos

1. Select oyster mushrooms with nicely shaped "fan-tails" and long stems. Set aside those smaller oyster mushroom bits to use as "eyes."
2. Brush a little olive oil on the bottom of baking dish with lid.
3. Mash tofu with fork. Add salt, onion powder and mix well.
4. Add flour to tofu mixture to absorb excess moisture.
5. Carefully put a handful (~1 T) tofu mixture to cover the entire stem of each oyster mushroom; squeeze and pack tight while shaping the body into a "fish" – narrow at the head with wider body gradually taper toward the tail end. Do not cover the "fan-tail." Gently lay it in the baking dish with its fan tail flat. Select dark brown mushroom bits as "eyes" @ the head.
6. Spray liquid aminos on the backs of each fish.
7. Cover and bake at 375°F for 15 minutes. Remove cover continue baking 10-15 minutes until firm and warm.

This is a fun way of serving tofu in a mock "fish" style. By combining two nutritious items (tofu, mushrooms), Mock Tofu Fish becomes an elegant dish.

Oyster mushrooms have been used as a culinary and medicinal ingredient. In Chinese medicine, oyster mushrooms are used as a tonic for the immune system. Mushrooms are high in protein, fiber and iron. Iron is essential for the growth of T lymphocytes - special cells that destroy viruses and tumor cells. Oyster mushrooms contain significant amounts of niacin which is important in repair damaged DNA.

Oyster mushrooms also contain ergothioneine, a unique antioxidant that protect the cells in the body, lower inflammation, and prevent the buildup of plaques in the arteries.

Tofu protects against heart disease and cancer. Tofu's isoflavones can reduce the risk of breast and prostate cancers, osteoporosis, and menopausal symptoms.

Marinated Gluten and Vegetables with Cashew Gravy

1 package of dehydrated gluten (or frozen tofu, tempeh, seitan)
2 carrots – sliced
2 celery stalks – sliced
1 small onion – sliced

Marinade Sauce:
½ cup warm water
1 T whole, unrefined sugar
¼ c Bragg Liquid Aminos
4–6 cloves garlic-minced
1 chili pepper – minced, optional

Cashew gravy:
1 c water
1 T raw cashews
1 T onion powder
½ t garlic powder
1T arrowroot powder or cornstarch
1T Bragg Liquid Aminos

1. Soak dehydrated gluten in water to soften. Squeeze out excess water. Cut to desired size and put in a large cooking pan.
2. Combine marinade ingredients in a bowl. Pour over the gluten and marinate for 30 minutes. Combine well.
3. Cook marinated gluten on low heat for 20 minutes or until most liquid is evaporated.
4. Place gravy ingredients in a blender and process until smooth. Pour into a small saucepan and cook over low heat until thickened. Stir frequently, add water if too thick.
5. In a large skillet sauté in small amount of water, carrots, celery, and onions until tender. Combine cooked gluten and vegetables with cashew-gravy.

Tofu Steaks with Tomatoes and Chestnuts

1 container of firm tofu (14-16 oz.)
3 cloves garlic – minced
1 t fresh ginger – minced
1 c diced tomatoes (canned or fresh)
1 c chestnuts – cooked or roasted
1 t onion powder
1 t salt or to taste
½ t dried sweet basil or handful fresh basil – chopped
Garnish with cilantro or fresh basil

1. Wrap firm tofu in clean towel to remove excess moisture.
2. Slice into steak-like slabs (4 thick or 8 thin slices).
3. "Fry" in a non-stick fry pan over medium heat until tofu slices turn golden brown on both sides. Remove. Keep warm.
4. Place garlic, ginger, diced tomatoes, chestnuts, onion powder, salt and basil in same pan cook over low heat until flavor is blended. If too dry, add a little water.
5. Arrange Tofu Steaks on serving platter top with tomato-chestnut sauce. Garnish with cilantro or fresh basil leaves.

Tofu adapts well with any flavor you wish to create. This dish blends a mixture of cultural flavors. The ingredients in this recipe contain cancer-fighting antioxidants and anti-inflammatory properties. I have included chestnuts for its alkaline benefits as most nuts are acidic. Chestnuts also protect the heart and combat cancer.

Marinated Tofu Cutlets with Asparagus Sauce

2 containers of medium-firm tofu (14 –16 oz.)
3 T Bragg Liquid Aminos
2 T water
2 T ketchup (Organic Ville Ketchup with agave)
1 t salt or to taste
1 package frozen asparagus (12 oz.) or fresh
½ c raw spinach leaves
1 green onion – chopped
½ c water or broth from asparagus
1/8 t salt or taste
Red bell peppers – chopped for garnish

To make the Tofu Cutlets:
1. Wrap tofu in clean kitchen towels to move excess moisture.
2. Slice to 4 slices per container and marinate in liquid aminos, water, ketchup, and salt for 30 minutes or longer.
3. Put the tofu and marinade in the flat pan and simmer with the cover on. Flip to other side, take off lid and simmer until sauce is cooked down.

To make the Asparagus Sauce:
1. Cook asparagus. Cut asparagus tips – reserve for garnish.
2. Blend asparagus, spinach, green onions, water (asparagus broth) and salt in a blender until creamy and smooth.

To serve: Spread Asparagus Sauce on serving platter, place Tofu Cutlets on top of Sauce. Garnish with asparagus tips and red bell peppers. Serve remaining Asparagus Sauce in a dish on the side.

Those who consumed tofu once a week or less were three times likely to contract prostate cancer than those who ate tofu daily. One 4 ounce serving of tofu packs 18 percent of adult's daily protein requirement, one-third of the daily requirement of iron, and an abundant supply of antioxidants. Antioxidants are believed to fend off cancers by protecting the DNA.

Asparagus contains flavonoids that inhibit the growth of cancer cells. Eating asparagus may help protect against cancers such as ovarian cancer, breast, colon, larynx, lung, and bone cancer.

Baked Tofu with Veggies

2 boxes tofu – slice length-wise through top center; then 6 slices cross-wise (total of 12 slices per box)
3 T Bragg Liquid Aminos
2 T Bill's Best Chik'nish powder
1 red onion – chopped
6 garlic cloves – crushed
2 celery stalks – chopped
6 mini bell peppers (all colors) – sliced
1 t onion powder
½ t salt or to taste
½ c green onions – chopped
½ c cilantro – chopped
2 T black sesame seeds

1. In a small dish mix liquid aminos and Chik'nish powder.
2. Place tofu slices on a non-stick baking pan or Silpat non-stick mat. Slowly drizzle liquid amino-mixture over tofu slices. Bake at 400°F for ~15 minutes on each side until golden brown.
3. Sauté onions and garlic in little water in the skillet until fragrant. Add celery, bell peppers and seasoning. Cook until vegetables are tender. Stir in green onions, cilantro and black sesame seeds.
4. Place baked tofu slices on serving platter. Top with veggies.

Regular tofu consumption can lead up to a 30 percent drop in cholesterol. One serving of tofu contains 18 percent of adult's daily protein requirement; one-third of the requirement of iron, and 10 percent of daily value for calcium. Tofu contains antioxidants (manganese, copper, and selenium) that protects against cancers.

Curried Potato –Vegetable Medley

1 medium onion – chopped
½ red onion – sliced
3 cloves garlic – minced
5 russet potatoes – cut into chunks with skin on
2 celery stalks – sliced
2 carrots – cut into rounds
2 T curry powder
1 t turmeric powder
3 c cooked or canned red, kidney, black or garbanzo beans – drained
3 fresh tomatoes – diced or 1 ½ c canned dice tomatoes, no juice
1 ½ cup water or broth (or cereal gruel for a thicker consistency)
½ t salt or to taste
Cayenne powder to taste, optional
1 green bell pepper – diced or ½ c frozen peas for garnish

1. In a large skillet, sauté onions until brown on medium heat.
2. Stir in potatoes celery, carrots, garlic, curry powder, and turmeric powder. Cook for 5 minutes.
3. Add beans, tomatoes, water, salt and cayenne, if using.
4. Cover and simmer on low until vegetables are done, about 45 minutes. Stir occasionally. Add green bell pepper or peas toward end of cooking, do not cover.

This dish serves as a one dish meal that packs with nutrition and taste. All the ingredients in this colorful medley provide an abundant supply of phytochemicals. Beans are rich in protein, vitamins, minerals, antioxidants, and fiber. Studies have found that tomatoes are protective against risks of a variety of cancers including colorectal, breast, prostate, lung and pancreatic cancer.

"Soy Steak" Jerky

Yield: ~60 pieces

1 package Vegan Steaks (Vege USA, product of Taiwan)

Marinade:
½ cup warm water
3 T unrefined sugar
1 T onion powder
5 T Bragg Liquid Aminos
6 red chili peppers – finely minced with seeds
1 t salt
1 T brown sesame seeds or flaxseeds
1 t five-spice powder (Asian markets)
1 T cornstarch in ¼ cup cold water
½ c beet water (cook beets, use the red beet broth for color)

1. Soak Vegan Steaks in water to soften. Squeeze excess water.
2. Cut each steak in half, and slice the halves horizontally into two thin halves for a total of four slices. Put in a large pan with lid.
3. In a bowl mix all ingredients for the marinade. Pour marinade over the vegan steaks; making sure each steak is saturated with the marinade.
4. Cover with lid cook over low heat for 30-40 minutes. Add water as needed to prevent scorching. Stir gently.
5. Place the cooked steaks on dehydrator trays lined with teflex sheets at 115°F for about 5 hours (less time, if prefer a softer-moist texture) or until dry on both sides (flip over midway). For a drier and chewier texture, you may need to remove the teflex sheets and continue dehydrating on mesh screens during the last hour, but do not allow them to become too dry.

Variation:

1. Use less red chili peppers for a less spicy version.

2. For curry-chicken-like flavor, omit chili peppers and beet water. Add extra ½ cup water, ½ t curry powder and 2 t Bill's Best Chik'nish powder.
3. For plain jerky flavor, omit chili peppers, five-spice powder and curry powder. You can add Bill's Best Chik'Nish powder if you wish.

The Soy Steak Jerky makes a lovely cold-platter. This recipe is low fat, no cholesterol, high fiber, rich in protein and minerals along with anti-cancer onions and chili peppers that can boost the immune system and increase the blood circulation. The unprocessed whole sugar gives a hint of molasses and vitamins, minerals and trace elements naturally found in the unrefined sugar cane.

Baked Shiitake Mushrooms and Onions

8 –10 shiitake mushroom caps
Mushroom stems – chopped
1 red onion – sliced
2 yellow onions – sliced
1–2 t Balsamic vinegar to taste
Sprays of Bragg Liquid Aminos

1. In a baking dish, place mushroom caps and brush with Balsamic vinegar in each cap.
2. Top with red and yellow onions slices. Spray liquid aminos over the onions and mushroom caps.
3. Scatter chopped mushroom stems over the mushrooms and onions.
4. Put a small amount of water (2 T) in bottom of baking dish. Cover and "steam-bake" at 250°F for 2 hours or until mushrooms are tender.

The Baked Mushrooms and Onions can be served as a main course. The longer it is baked the onions and mushrooms seem to taste sweeter.

The shiitake mushrooms have a strong antiviral effect due to the interferons inherent in the mushrooms. Interferons are natural proteins in the mushrooms that boost the immune system. Shiitake mushrooms contain all the essential amino acids in a better ratio than meat, milk or eggs. Consumption of shiitake mushrooms can also help lower cholesterol levels by up to 40 – 45 percent.

Portobello Mushroom Steaks and Sweet Onions

3 Portobello mushrooms – stemmed
Mushroom stems – chopped
4-5 cloves garlic – minced
2 T Bragg Liquid Aminos
1 T water
½ t Balsamic vinegar
1 sweet onion – sliced
¼ t salt to taste
3 c arugula

1. Gently remove stems and clean mushrooms. Put on a plate.
2. Mix garlic, liquid aminos, water, and vinegar in a bowl.
3. Pour the sauce into the caps of mushrooms. Let marinate. Put in refrigerator to marinate longer, if not cooking right away.
4. Sauté onions in a dry skillet pan over medium high heat to caramelize until brown. Stir. Add 1 tsp. water or more to loosen caramelized onions. Add salt. Set aside.
5. In the same skillet pan over low heat place marinated mushroom caps and stems; cook for 8-10 minutes until tender. If needed add one tablespoon water at a time, continue simmer with lid on.
6. Spread arugula on a platter. Place the mushrooms cap-side down over the greens. Top with the sweet onions. Drizzle with Balsamic vinegar if desire.

The Portobello mushrooms often spell as portabellas. They are the larger version of the button or crimini mushrooms. Their texture is chewier and denser; often used as meat substitute.

One cup of Portobello mushrooms provides 5 grams of protein and 3 grams of fiber. They are naturally low in sodium, but high in minerals and vitamins. One cup also provides 31 percent of the daily requirement for selenium, an antioxidant mineral that protects healthy cells from free radical damages, and repairs the damaged cells. The Portobello mushrooms have an extremely high rating for its antioxidant capabilities. More antioxidants are found in the caps than in the stems. Unlike many other foods, most of the antioxidants are not destroyed by cooking.

Onions are rich in flavonoids that are protective against cancers. Flavonoids in onion tend to be more concentrated in the outer layers of the flesh. To maximize your health benefits, peel off as little of the fleshy edible portion as possible.

Arugula belongs to the cabbage family. They are useful for reducing risks of cancers. Three cups of arugula provide over 100 per cent of daily vitamin K needs. Vitamin K is known to promote bone health and brain function.

Portobello Mushrooms with Tofu-Ginger Sauce

1 box medium-firm tofu
½ cup water
2 T Bragg Liquid Aminos
1 inch ginger – chopped
2-3 Portobello mushrooms – sliced (stems chopped)
1 red onion – chopped
2 cloves garlic – chopped
½ t onion powder
¼ t salt
1 t oregano
½ c cilantro or green onions – chopped as garnish

1. Blend in a blender tofu, water, liquid aminos, and ginger until smooth.
2. Sauté onions and garlic in little water until translucent. Add mushrooms and sauté until soft with lid on. Add onion powder, salt to taste, and oregano.
3. Pour tofu-ginger sauce over mushrooms and combine well briefly. Turn off heat and stir in cilantro.

Rice and Bean Casserole

6 c cooked brown rice (black, red, sticky brown or combinations)
2 t Bill's Best Chik'nish Vegetarian Seasoning
1 c cooked red beans
1 c cooked black beans
½ onions chopped
2 c king oyster mushrooms or shiitake mushrooms – chopped
½ t salt
1T Bragg Liquid Aminos

1. In a large bowl combine cooked rice with Chik'nish seasoning until well mixed. Set aside.
2. In a separate bowl, coarsely mash the cooked red and black beans with a fork or briefly process in food processor.
3. Sauté onions and mushrooms. Add salt. Add mashed beans and liquid aminos. Mix well.
4. Place half of the cooked rice in the bottom of a casserole dish with lid. Place all the bean-mushroom mixture on top of rice. Put remaining half of the rice over the bean-mushrooms.
5. Bake at 325°F for 40 minutes with cover on until heated through. Serve with an ice cream scoop or small custard cup for round-mounds on plate if desire.

Rice serves as a staple food worldwide. Whole grain rice contains essential carbohydrates, B vitamins, vitamin E and minerals.

Beans' nutritional contributions have been overlooked. Just by eating legumes four times per week one can drop the heart disease (the number one killer) risk by 22 percent. Its antioxidants can keep normal cells from turning cancerous. Black beans are rich in folates essential for nervous system health. In addition, black beans are extremely rich source of molybdenum – useful for detoxifying sulfites. Studies also suggest that molybdenum deficiencies can result in impotence in older men. Moreover, all beans stabilizes blood sugar, prevents constipation and low cost.

Curry Tofu with Coconut Milk and Rice

Marinade:
2 t Bill's Best Chik'nish
½ t onion powder
¼ t garlic powder
½ t turmeric powder
¼ t cumin
1 t salt
½ cup water
1 medium firm tofu (14 oz.) – frozen, thawed, wrapped in towel
½ red onions – thinly sliced
3 c cooked brown rice
1/3 c organic raisins
½ c frozen peas
1 can (14 oz.) light coconut milk

1. Place marinade ingredients in a large bowl and set aside.
2. Cut tofu into small cubes (~1" cubes), add to marinade. If using until later, place in refrigerator.
3. Sauté onions in a large skillet on medium heat until brown and caramelized. Add marinated tofu cubes with little water if needed. Cook for 5 minutes.
4. Add cooked rice, raisins, and coconut milk. Reduce heat to low and simmer for 10 minutes, stir frequently and add more water as needed. Stir in peas, cook until tender - 5 minutes. Adjust salt to taste. Serve warm. Garnish with shredded toasted coconut if desired.

Tofu contains the soybean peptides that slow cancerous growth in laboratory studies. The researchers showed that soybean peptides slowed colon cancer cell growth by 73 percent, liver cancer cell growth by 70 percent, and lung cancer cell growth by 68 percent. Consuming more soy may help slash cancer risk in people according to researchers at the University of Arkansas.

Brown rice is high in fiber, an important nutrient that protects against colon cancer and breast cancer. Brown rice is high in manganese, important in fighting free radicals. One cup of brown rice contains 88 percent of the recommended daily value of manganese, and also rich in selenium which destroys cancer cells, repairs DNA, and enhances the immune system.

Raisins contain phenols that have potent antioxidant benefits that help to scavenge free radicals in the body. The seasonings in the marinade have anti-cancer properties. Curcumin, in turmeric can suppress cancer cells and stop them from spreading.

Mexi-Fritters with Corn Salsa

1 large red onions – finely chopped (save 2 T for Salsa)

2–3 poblano chili peppers – finely chopped (save ¼ c for Salsa)

1 ½ c canned or cooked pinto bean – drained

2 T water

1 T Bragg Liquid Aminos

1 T lemon juice

1 T arrowroot powder or cornstarch

1 T whole wheat flour

1 box firm tofu (14 oz.) drained and wrapped with kitchen towel

¼ c corn (frozen, thawed or canned, drained)

½ c cilantro – chopped

1 t salt

1/8 t cayenne powder, optional

1. In a large skillet, put chopped red onions and poblano chili with little water. Cover and cook over medium heat until soft.
2. Mash pinto beans with a fork. Set aside.
3. In a small bowl whisk together water, liquid aminos, lemon juice, arrowroot powder, and whole wheat flour.
4. Use hand to crumble tofu and add to the skillet with red onions and poblano chilies. Sauté until the mixture looks dry.
5. Stir in mashed beans, arrowroot liquid mixture, corn, cilantro, salt and cayenne if using. Cook briefly until well combined.
6. Drop small pin-pone-ball-size mounds unto non-stick baking sheets (yields approximately 20-24 patties). Flatten with back of spoon. Bake @ 450° F for 10-15 minutes or until firm.

Corn Salsa

2 T red onions – finely chopped
¼ c poblano chili – finely chopped
1 tomato – finely chopped, optional
1 T lemon juice or to taste
1 c corn (thawed if frozen)
¼ c cilantro – finely chopped
½ t salt to taste
Toss all ingredients together and serve over the Mexi-Fritters.

Pinto beans are an excellent source of protein and iron comparable to meat. The beans are rich in B vitamins which help with brain function, memory, and minerals useful for heart health. The fiber helps to control cholesterol levels, blood sugar fluctuations, improve digestion, and prevent constipation.

Tofu contributes calcium – a single serving delivers 10 percent of daily need for calcium. Onions and chili peppers combat cancer, boost immune system, and reduce risk of heart attack.

Tofu Sticks with Sweet and Sour Sauce   Serves 8

1 box firm tofu (14 oz.) – drained and wrapped with kitchen towel
2 T flax seed meal or 1 T flax seeds grind in coffee grinder
2 T arrowroot powder or corn starch
1 T liquid aminos or soy sauce
¼ cup water
2 brown rice cakes (or1 c rice cake meal)
1 T unbleached all-purpose flour
½ t turmeric powder
¼ t garlic powder
¼ t onion powder
¼ t paprika

1. Pulverize rice cakes into a fine meal in a blender. Set aside in a shallow dish.
2. In a second shallow bowl stir in flaxseed meal, arrowroot powder, liquid aminos, and water.
3. Combine dry ingredients (flour, turmeric, garlic, onion and paprika) with the rice cake meal.
4. Slice tofu into 16 sticks (8 slices then cut each slice into 2). Dip each tofu stick in liquid flaxseed meal mixture (shake off excess); then in rice cake mixture, coating all sides.
5. Place on a non-stick baking pan and bake at 350° F oven for 25 minutes. Turn over to other side and bake for 15 minutes to golden brown or desired crispiness.

Sweet and Sour Sauce   Yield: 1 ½ cup

1 c unsweetened pineapple juice
1 T Bragg Liquid Aminos or soy sauce
2 T ketchup made with agave nectar
2 T apple cider vinegar
1–2 t lemons juice or to desired tartness
1 T fresh grated ginger – optional
2 T arrowroot powder or cornstarch

1. Combine all ingredients in a small sauce pan over medium heat.
2. Bring to boil and let simmer on low until thickened. Add more
    water if the sauce becomes too thick. Stir frequently.

The Tofu Sticks can be made ahead of time and then just reheat for
few a minutes before serving. The Sweet and Sour Sauce can also be
made ahead and then serve at room temperature. For those with wheat
or gluten sensitivity, you can omit the flour.

Tofu supplies a full spectrum of nutrients that can protect us against
heart disease, diabetes, cancer, and age-related decline. Tofu provides
many phytonutrients with antioxidant and free radical-scavenging
benefits.

Flaxseeds are rich in antioxidants protecting the heart, Alzheimer's
disease, and macular degeneration.

Brown rice is rich in manganese, a nutrient important in fighting
free radicals. It also provides selenium, an antioxidant.

Turmeric has strong anti-inflammatory and antioxidant properties
and may prevent and slow the progression of Alzheimer's disease by
removing amyloid build up in the brain. This spice also contains anti-
cancer activity, and it can stop the growth of new blood vessels in
tumors.

Garlic, onions and paprika are known for their antioxidant
properties. These spices protect our cells from free radical damages.

Red Bean and Mushroom Meat Loaf

1 c cooked or canned red beans – partially mashed with fork
¼ c dehydrated soy bits – rehydrate with little water
½ c cooked brown rice
2 T uncooked quinoa – rinse well with water
½ c onions – chopped
1 c button mushrooms – chopped
½ c green bell peppers – chopped
1 T nutritional yeast
¼ t sage
1 t Bragg Liquid Aminos
Salt to taste

1. In a bowl mix the cooked beans, soy or gluten bits, cooked rice, and rinsed quinoa.
2. Place 2 T water in skillet over medium-low heat, sauté onions, mushrooms, green bell peppers, yeast, sage, and liquid aminos.
3. Add the rice and bean mixture to the mushroom mixture. Adjust salt to taste.
4. Place in a small baking dish with cover or a non-stick mini-loaf-bread-pan cover with foil.
5. Bake at 350°F for 10 minutes with cover. Then reduce heat to 325°F continue baking for 20 minutes or until done (can take off cover during the last 10 minutes). Carefully using butter knife to loosen the edges of the loaf and turn over unto a platter. Gently cut into slices and serve.

Red beans are rich in protein, iron, and the B vitamins. It rates the highest in antioxidants. Whole beans, brown rice and mushrooms all combat cancer, stabilize blood sugar, lower cholesterol, and prevent constipation. Quinoa was named the "mother of all grains." It provides complete protein, and rich in minerals.

Mushrooms are loaded with the nutrients for our bodies to generate energy and repair cells. They are rich in digestive enzymes, vitamins, minerals, protein and vitamin D2. White mushrooms also protect against inflammation. Chronic inflammation increases the risks of type 2 diabetes, cardiovascular disease, and cancers.

Rice Wraps

1 package (25 sheets) rice wraps (sold in most Asian markets)
1 firm tofu or Bowtie Kelp with Soy Curls (see recipe Main Dishes)
Kale Kraut Salad (see recipe Salads)
1 red bell pepper – sliced into thin strips
1 cucumber – sliced into thin strips
½ package beans sprouts – rinsed and drained
1 avocado – sliced
2 c wood ear mushrooms, optional (sold in Asian markets)
2 green onions – chopped, optional
½ c ground peanuts, optional

1. Crumble tofu or Bowtie Kelp with Soy Curls. Set aside.
2. Prepare Kale Kraut Salad and set side.
3. Soak wood mushrooms, if using, and take out the tough center stem. Boil for 5 minutes in water until tender. Drain and season with liquid aminos or salt to taste. Chill.
4. To assemble: soak each dried-rice-sheet momentarily in a shallow container large enough to submerse the entire rice sheet in room temperature water; quickly place it on a plate. Then add the prepared ingredients according to the order listed above. Wrap it up like a burrito. Serve.

A fun way to serve the Rice Wraps is to have each person to customize his or her own wrap. Although the rice wraps are made from white rice which is poor nutritionally: however, the ingredients for the stuffing are nutritious. For a healthier version, one can use the whole wheat pocket breads, split into two single layers.

The Chinese have been growing mung bean sprouts for 3000 years. Mung beans contain compounds that inhibit the formation and growth of cancerous tumors. The sprouts provide dietary fiber which can protect against colon cancer and breast cancer. The sprouts are high in protein, vitamins, minerals, and high in live enzymes.

The wood ear mushrooms provide 18 percent protein and 50 percent fiber. They have anticancer, anti-inflammatory, and cardio-protective properties that help to prevent cancer, stroke and heart disease. The wood ear mushrooms provide a good source of calcium, containing twice the amount of calcium compared to milk. It is also rich in iron – seven times more than pig liver.

The red bell peppers contain powerful antioxidants for the prevention of cancers such as stomach, colon, breast, prostate, and lung cancer. Red bell peppers are packed with vitamin C – the richest source of all fruits and vegetables.

Cabbage Rolls

8 large cabbage leaves (or12 smaller leaves)
1 c dehydrated soy curls (www.butlerfoods.com)

Marinade:
½ cup warm water
2 T Bragg Liquid Aminos
2 cloves garlic – minced
1 T ginger – minced
1 t onion powder
1–2 shakes dried crushed red pepper, optional

Stuffing:
1 carrot – thinly sliced into match sticks
4 mushrooms – sliced
2 green onions – chopped
½ cucumber - sliced into thin strips
½ red bell pepper – sliced into thin strips
White miso paste, optional

1. Marinate the dehydrated soy curls in marinade for 15 minutes.
2. Carefully trim off hard veins from large cabbage leaves while keeping the leaves intact. Bring water to boil in a large pot, gently place 1 or 2 cabbage leaves to simmer for 5 minutes until soft. Set aside on plate.
3. Put 2 T water in a skillet, sauté over medium heat carrots, marinated soy curls, and mushrooms until cooked, 7-8 minutes; add little water as needed. Add green onions.
4. To make cabbage rolls:
   a. Carefully using butter knife spread a thin layer of miso paste over the lower half of cabbage leaf.
   b. Place ~2 T stuffing (1 T on small leaves) at the lower stem- end of the cabbage leaf. Put cucumber and red bell pepper slices on top of stuffing.

5. Wrap the stuffing and raw veggies and roll toward the top of the leaf tug in sides making sure stuffing stays inside. Place the seam face down on the plate.

6. Using a sharp knife, carefully slice the cabbage roll diagonally into two rolls. Enjoy.

Instead of the marinated soy curls, you can substitute pressed tofu slices or gluten slices. Once you have all the ingredients cut, the assembling of the Cabbage Rolls is quick and easy. For children, you may wish to use the smaller leaves with less stuffing.

Cabbage belongs to the cruciferous family that combats cancer by detoxify toxic chemicals, and arrest growth of cancer cells.

Stuffed Eggplant

4-6 Japanese eggplants

Stuffing:
½ c onions – finely chopped
5 garlic cloves – minced
1 T fresh ginger – finely chopped
1 c cooked or canned beans – drained and mashed with fork
Insides of cooked eggplants – finely chopped
¼ c canned or fresh tomatoes –finely chopped
¼ cup corn – thawed if frozen
½ c green bell pepper – finely chopped
1 t Bragg Liquid Aminos
½ t salt to taste
2–3 shakes cayenne powder to taste, optional
Red chili pepper flakes, optional for garnish

Gravy:
1 T arrowroot powder or cornstarch
¾ cup water
1–2 T Bragg Liquid Aminos

1. Bring water to boil with 1 t salt in a large pan. Put in whole eggplants and cook until soft about 10 minutes.
2. In a small bowl, mix the gravy ingredients and set aside.
3. When cool, slice eggplants in ½ length-wise. Carefully scoop out insides and chop to small pieces; set aside. Place eggplant shells in a baking pan with lid.
4. To make the stuffing: sauté onions in skillet on medium heat until brown. Stir in garlic, ginger, and mashed beans. Turn heat to low, add chopped eggplants, tomatoes and corn until soft. Add little water if needed. Add liquid aminos, salt, and cayenne if using. Stir occasionally. Turn off heat.
5. Add green bell peppers and mix well.

6. Fill eggplant shells with stuffing. Pour gravy over eggplants. Sprinkle with red chili pepper flakes, if desire.
7. Pour a little water at bottom of baking pan. Cover and "Steam-Bake" at 400° F for 15-20 minutes until warm.

You can use any beans for this recipe - kidney beans, white bean or garbanzos. This dish can be prepared earlier; then bake it just before serving.

We find that the colorful fruits and vegetables provide an abundance of health-protective phytonutrients. The blue and purple eggplant contains the anti-inflammatory and antioxidant anthocyanin that combats cancer, prevents heart disease, reverses aging, and sharpens the brain. Other blue and purple plant foods include purple bell peppers, purple yams, purple cauliflower, red or purple cabbage, plum, blackberries, blueberries, and grapes.

Tomatoes are known for its lycopene, a carotenoid with health benefits. But tomatoes also contain other protective phytonutrients that work in synergy with each other.

Soy Bean-curd Sticks

2 (6-oz.) packages dried soy bean-curd sticks (Asian markets)

Sauce:
¼ cup Bragg Liquid Aminos
2 T garlic powder
4 T nutritional yeast
½ c to 1 c water

1. In a long pan with sides, soak the bean-curd sticks in water until soft. Discard the soaked water. Cut into 3–4 inch pieces and put back in the tray. If the sticks appear tough, put in a pan cover with water and briefly boil until soft. Drain water.
2. Pour sauce over the soaked sticks.
3. Place marinated sticks in single layer in flat bottom skillet on low heat. Pour part of the sauce over the sticks. Cover to simmer until tender. Uncover, turnover and briefly brown the other side until most liquid is absorbed, and the bean-curd sticks are thoroughly cooked.

Garnish with green onions or cilantro. Bean-curd sticks can be served either hot or cold. They freeze well.

Soybeans are now staple foods around the world. Soybeans contain all essential amino acids, fatty acids, minerals, vitamins, phytonutrients, and fiber. Epidemiological studies have found soy foods reduce risks for cancers of breast, colon, and prostate.

Singapore Mock Chicken

1 package (6 oz.) dried soy bean-curd sticks
1 package (8 oz.) baby Bella or Crimini mushrooms – sliced
3 stalks green onions – sliced
½ t ground cumin
½ t turmeric
1 T Bragg Liquid Aminos
1 T nutritional yeast
Sprinkle dried crushed red pepper or 1/8 t cayenne powder
Cilantro leaves for garnish

1. Soak dried bean-curd sticks in water until soft. Discard soaking water.
2. Cut into ~ 2– 3 inch lengths. Place in a large pan. Cover with fresh water and cook over medium heat until cooked. Some sticks may become shapeless pieces. Drain excess water. Set aside.
3. In a skillet, sauté mushrooms and green onions. Add salt to taste. Dish up and set aside.
4. In the same skillet sauté drained cooked soybean curd sticks along with broken shapeless pieces. Add cumin, turmeric, liquid aminos, nutritional yeast, and dried crushed red pepper. Mix until flavors are well blended.
5. Stir in mushroom mixture and combine briefly. Serve on platter. Garnish with cilantro leaves.

The Singapore Mock Chicken show case the versatility of the soy bean-curd in Asian cuisine. You can modify the soy bean-curd by using different seasonings and by adding variety of vegetables.

Crimini mushrooms in the diet can help prevent over production of pro-inflammatory molecules. Most chronic diseases are due to inflammation. Mushrooms are also rich in selenium, an antioxidant that protects our healthy cells from free radical damage.

Soy Bean-curd Mock Duck

2 (6 oz.) packages of dried soy bean-curd sheets

Sauce:
1 c filtered water
¼ c Bragg Liquid Aminos
1 t onion powder
1 t garlic powder
1 t Bill's Chik 'nish, optional
1 T + 1 t arrowroot powder

1. Place bean-curd sheets in a long pan with sides. Soak in water until soft. Drain water.
2. In a bowl mix filtered water, liquid aminos, onion powder, garlic powder, Chick'nish if using, and arrowroot powder. Mix well.
3. Pour sauce over the bean-curd sheets.
4. Roll up each sheet into burrito-like flat log, and marinate in the sauce to allow flavor to soak through.
5. Place 4 to 5 logs into a flat bottom skillet with lid. Pour some sauce over the logs.
6. Simmer on low, cook slowly with cover on.
7. Carefully turn over the logs, add more water as needed. Continue to simmer until most of the liquid is absorbed and the logs are thoroughly cooked.
8. When cooled, slice each log into 7 to 8 slices cross-wise.

The Soy Bean-curd Mock Duck can be served as a main entrée either warm or cold. It freezes well. Some Asian markets may carry the fresh soy bean-curd sheets in the refrigerated section. When using the fresh sheets, you do not need to pre-soak them. Just marinate directly in the sauce.

Soybeans need to play a prominent role in the diet for everyone. Those who consume more soy generally have lower rates of colon cancer, breast cancer, and prostate cancer. In countries with higher meat consumption, cancers are much more prevalent than areas where diets are predominately plant-based.

Taro Root "Drum Sticks"

4 taro root
4 dried bean-curd sheets – soften and cut into triangles (~6" X 7")
1 T whole wheat flour or whole wheat pastry flour
1-2 T Bragg Liquid Aminos
1 t onion powder
½ t garlic powder
¼ t honey, or maple syrup or agave nectar
2 T water to make a medium thick paste

1. Boil taro root until done (~20 minutes), gently peel the skin.
2. In a bowl mix the flour, liquid aminos, onion powder, garlic powder, sweetener, and water to make a medium thick paste.
3. In a shallow container soften the bean-curd sheets in lukewarm water. Cut to size. Place on empty plate.
4. Spread a thin layer of paste on the bean-curd sheet.
5. Coat the taro root in the paste* and place the coated taro root at one corner of the bean-curd sheet. Roll up as you tuck in other corners into a drum-stick like "thigh." Seal the edges with paste.
6. Place in a baking dish and spray a mist of liquid aminos on top of each drum-stick. Put a little water (~1/4 c) at bottom of baking pan.
7. Steam - Bake at 400°F with cover on for 15-20 minutes until heated through. If you prefer a crispier skin, take cover off and bake additional few minutes until golden brown.

*An alternative method is: Mash the taro root with a fork. Season with 1 T onion powder and ½ t salt (you can also add mixed vegetables as corn, carrots and/or peas). Spread the paste over the entire bean-curd sheet. Place seasoned mashed taro-mixture in one corner of the bean-curd sheet; wrap it into a "thigh" drum stick shape.

To imitate chicken-like drum sticks, select taro roots that look like chicken thighs. The soy bean-curd sheets take on the appearance and texture of chicken skin; of course minus all the cholesterol and toxins.

You can cut the bean-curd sheets to a size that will wrap snugly the taro roots.

Taro roots are high in fiber and nutrition. They minimize the risks for heart attack, hypertension, colon cancer, and kidney disease. Taro roots aid in digestion and improve immune functions.

A word about sulfites: Sulfites have been used since 1660's as preservatives because of their antibacterial, antioxidant, and anti-browning properties. They are added to a variety of foods to prevent spoilage. Sulfites are found in many foods including the dried soy bean-curd sticks and sheets plus many other food and beverage products.

However, some individuals may have sulfite sensitivity. Be sure to read labels for sulfite containing compounds (sodium metabisulfite, sodium hydrosulfite, sulfites). The vast majority of adverse events related to sulfites usually occur in those with asthma. The chemical compounds are readily soluble in water. It is best to soak the soy bean-curd sticks and sheets in water, drain, then use filtered water to cook them.

Spaghetti with Edamame Sauce

8 oz. (1/2 pound) spaghetti
1 medium onion – chopped
4 cloves garlic – chopped
1 c canned tomatoes or 3 fresh tomatoes – chopped
1 – 1 ½ c tomato juice or water
2 T organic ketchup, no refined sugar
½ t salt or to taste
1 T Bragg Liquid Aminos
2 T nutritional yeast flakes
¼ t dried oregano
¼ t dried basil
½ t unrefined sugar
1 c cooked edamame or peas

1. Cook spaghetti according to package direction.
2. In a skillet, put ¼ cup water over medium heat. When bubbly, add onions and garlic, sauté until soft.
3. Add chopped tomatoes and liquids, simmer on low.
4. Add ketchup, salt, liquid aminos, nutritional yeast, oregano, basil, and unrefined sugar.
5. Stir in cooked edamame or peas.
6. Mix cooked rinsed spaghetti with sauce. Serve while hot.

Nutritional yeast is a non-active form of yeast that adds a delicious nutty flavor to food. It contains 18 amino acids, 15 minerals, and rich in B-complex vitamins including B-12. Regular consumption of nutritional yeast can improve immune response, reduce cholesterol, control blood sugar levels, and enhance anti-cancer properties.

Eggplant, Sundried Tomatoes, Spinach, Edamame with Fusilli Pasta

1 lb. Fusilli pasta
5 cloves garlic – minced
2 chili peppers – minced, optional
1 eggplant – diced with skin on
10 whole slices of sundried tomatoes – soaked with water to cover (save liquid) and sliced
1 t salt or to taste
1 T Bragg Liquid Aminos
1 package (6 oz.) of baby spinach – chopped or one bunch fresh
1 c fresh tomatoes – diced
1 t dried oregano
2 t apple cider vinegar
1 c cooked edamame

1. Cook pasta according to package direction. Drain and reserve 3/4 c pasta-cooking water.
2. Place 2 T water in skillet over medium heat. Add garlic, chili peppers. Stir briefly and add eggplant. Cook for 5 minutes. Stir and add water as needed to cook eggplant.
3. Add sundried tomatoes and soaking liquid. Continue to cook until eggplant and sundried tomatoes are tender (add more water if needed). Add salt and liquid aminos to taste.
4. Add tomatoes, spinach, oregano, apple cider vinegar, edamame and pasta with reserved pasta-cooking water. Combine until spinach wilts and pasta thoroughly heated.

Whole Grain Penne with Eggplant, Tomatoes, and Olives

2 red bell peppers – chopped
6 garlic cloves – chopped
½ t dried crushed red pepper
1 large eggplant – cut into ½ inch cubes with skin on
1 T dried oregano
1 28-oz. can diced tomatoes in juice
½ c fresh basil – chopped
½ c black or green olives – sliced
1 t lemon juice
¼ t salt or to taste
1 T Bragg Liquid Aminos
1 box (12 oz.) whole grain penne pasta

Topping – combine ingredients in a small bowl:
½ c ground raw cashews – grind in coffee grinder or blender
2 T nutritional yeast
¼ t pasta seasoning blend, optional

1. Sauté over medium heat bell peppers, garlic, and crushed pepper in little water until fragrant.
2. Add eggplant and oregano. Reduce heat to low; add ¼ – ½ c water as needed to cook the eggplant. Cover and cook until eggplant softens, about 10 minutes. Stir occasionally.
3. Add tomatoes with juice, basil, olives, and lemon juice. Cover and simmer until all vegetables are tender, about 15 minutes. Season it with salt to taste.
4. Cook penne pasta according to package direction until just tender, but still firm. Drain. Combine pasta with vegetable mixture. Mix in liquid aminos. Transfer to baking dish. Sprinkle cashew topping over pasta and cover.
5. Preheat oven to 350°F. Bake pasta for about 25 minutes until heated through (40 minutes if refrigerated). Take off cover and

bake additional 5 minutes for a golden color. For a chewier crust, bake few more minutes. Garnish with basil.

Most pasta dishes call for lots of cheese and oil. This is a healthier version. For additional flavor and moisture, add a jar of Trader Joe's spaghetti sauce (no sugar).

Eggplants contain phytonutrients that protect cells against harmful damages from free radicals. Tomatoes are known for its lycopene, a carotenoid with many health benefits particularly against a variety of cancers.

Garbanzo Sauce over Pasta Noodles

2 c cooked or canned garbanzo beans (chickpeas)*
1 can diced tomatoes
1 medium onion – chopped
5 cloves of garlic – chopped
1 t onion powder
1 t nutritional yeast flakes
½ t dried basil
½ t dried oregano
¼ t salt
¼ t paprika
1 package pasta noodles

1. Put all ingredients (except pasta) in saucepan simmer on low for 1 hour.
2. Cook pasta noodles according to package direction.
3. Pour Garbanzo Sauce over pasta noodles just before serving.

*For a creamier sauce, blend half of the garbanzo beans in the blender until smooth before cooking the sauce.

Besides using this recipe over pasta noodles, the Garbanzo Sauce also goes well with cooked brown rice.

The beans are rich in protein, fiber, calcium and iron. Garbanzos are loaded with the trace mineral manganese necessary for strong bones. One cup of garbanzos will provided over 84 percent of the recommended daily requirement. Garbanzo beans are rich in tryptophan, an essential amino acid that is a precursor to serotonin. Serotonin regulates both mood and sleep.

Tomatoes contain a variety of protective phytonutrients that work in synergy with each other. Tomatoes are protective against risks of certain cancers such as lung, stomach, prostate, colorectal, breast, endometrial, and pancreatic cancers.

Bowtie Kelp with Soy Curls

4 cups of bowtie kelp (~1.5 pounds)
½ cup warm water
1 T unrefined sugar
1 T Bragg Liquid Aminos
4 cloves garlic – minced
1 chili pepper – minced

To make Soy Curls:
2 c dehydrated soy curls (www.butlerfoods.com) - in 1 c warm water
1 T garlic powder
1 t Bill's Best Chik'nish Vegetarian Seasoning
Shake of Cayenne powder – optional
Cilantro – chopped for garnish, optional

1. Put first 6 ingredients in a sauce pan over medium heat until boil; continue to simmer on low heat until tender, approximately 40 minutes. Add more water as needed.
2. In a skillet with 2 T water on medium heat, sauté rehydrated Soy Curls. Add seasonings and simmer with cover on until tender about 10-15 minutes.
3. Combine cooked Bowtie Kelp with Soy Curls. Garnish with cilantro and serve

For variation, I add some cooked green beans or carrots or any vegetable you wish to this dish. Instead of the Bowtie Kelp, you can use other types of sea vegetables that most Asian markets carry. The Soy Curls are made from whole soy beans that provide not only a meaty texture, but also all the goodness found in the soy beans.

Seaweed or sea vegetables is the common name for about 10,000 known species of the marine plants. They are divided into three types according to their color: brown, red and green. Seaweed contains significant amounts of vitamins and also trace-amounts of all the amino acids. They offer one of the broadest ranges of minerals of any food, containing virtually all the minerals found in the ocean – many of the same minerals found in human blood. Sea vegetables have anti-inflammatory benefits, anti-viral activity and anti-cancer properties. Sea vegetables can decrease the risk for breast cancer and colon cancer. The most common edible seaweeds are:

Kelp – light brown to dark green
Nori – purple-black to green
Hijiki – small strands of black wiry pasta like
Kombu – dark color, sold in strips or sheets
Wakame – similar to kombu, used to make miso soup
Arame – lacy, wiry sea vegetable with a sweet and milder taste
Dulse – soft, chewy texture, reddish-brown color

Butternut Squash Shepherd's Pie

Stuffing:
1 butternut squash – chopped to ½" cubes
1 large sweet onions – chopped
2 garlic – minced
2 c cook garbanzos
1 green bell peppers – chopped
2 T whole wheat flour in 1/3 c water
1 t Bill's Best Chik'nish Vegetarian Seasoning
½ t salt

Top Crust:
10–12 cooked and peeled potatoes
1 T white miso paste in 1 T water
1 t salt
1 small red bell peppers – chopped fine as garnish

1. Peel butternut squash using a vegetable peeler to the orange flesh. Cut into small cubes.
2. Place 2 T water in a large skillet over medium heat, sauté onions until fragrant; add garlic. Reduce heat, add butternut squash, cover and cook until soft. If too dry, add tiny bit of water.
3. Mix water, flour and seasonings in a small bowl. Set aside.
4. Add cooked garbanzos and green bell pepper to the butternut mixture in the skillet. Stir in flour and seasonings cook until mixture thickens.
5. Spread butternut stuffing in a baking dish (9" X 13").
6. Mash cooked potatoes with miso paste and salt to taste.
7. Spread mashed potatoes over the butternut squash. Smooth with back of spoon. Use a fork, make wavy ridges on top. Bake at 375°F for 30 minutes. Garnish with red bell peppers.

Butternut squash is a nutrition star. It is low in fat, but rich in vitamins, minerals and fiber. Butternut squash provides nearly three-hundred percent of the daily recommended value of vitamin A, component of every cell. This vegetable is also rich in vitamin C, an antioxidant that can prevent certain kinds of cancer, and keep the immune system working properly. One cup of butternut squash provides 50 percent of daily recommended value of vitamin C.

Twice Baked Potatoes with Sunflower Seeds and Herbs

4 large baking potatoes
½ c raw cashews – soaked and drained
3 T nutritional yeast
1 T lemon juice or 1 T apple cider vinegar
1 T white miso paste
2 T water
½ c chives – finely chopped, divided
½ c cilantro or parsley – finely chopped, divided
1/3 c raw sunflower seeds – coarsely grounded, divided
¼ c unsweetened shredded coconuts

1. Bake potatoes @ 400°F for 1 hour or until soft to squeeze.
2. Process the cashews, nutritional yeast, lemon juice, miso paste and water in food processor until smooth. Transfer to a large bowl.
3. Gently slice off top of potato lengthwise. Carefully scoop out flesh into the cashew mixture leave ¼-inch thickness near skin to keep shell intact. Place the shells on a baking sheet.
4. Combine the cashew mixture with the potato flesh. Add half of the chives, cilantro (parsley) and sunflower seeds. Season it with salt to taste.
5. Equally divide the mixture among the potato shells and bake 15 minutes until tops turn golden brown.
6. Garnish with remaining chives, cilantro and sunflower seeds.

The Twice Baked Potatoes are scrumptious and a very healthy low-calorie and high fiber food. Potatoes contain phytochemicals including flavonoids and a recently identified compound called kukoamine that appears to help to lower blood pressure. Potatoes are rich in B vitamins, vitamin C, and minerals.

Cashews contain mono-unsaturated fats, rich in omega-3-fatty acids, and vitamin E. Cashews have proanthocyanidins (a class of flavonols) that actually starve tumors and stop cancer cells from dividing. Cashews contain copper that can eliminate free radicals.

Sunflower seeds prevent cholesterol buildup and have anti-inflammatory properties. Sunflower seeds are rich in vitamin E, one of the best sources of antioxidants that can reduce free radical damages. Sunflower seeds also contain selenium that promotes the repair of DNA which helps in the prevention of cancer. In addition, selenium promotes the removal and disintegration of old cancerous body cells. The seeds are rich in folates (B vitamin) that can promote the formation of new blood cells, improve our oxygen–carrying capacity and immunity.

Mexi-Potatoes with Baby Bella and Guacamole

4 baked potatoes

Stuffing:
½ c onions – chopped
3 cloves garlic – chopped
1 c fresh baby Bella mushrooms – sliced
1/8 t salt

Topping:
1 avocado – finely diced
1 tomato – finely diced
2 T raw walnuts – finely diced
½ t lemon juice
2 T cilantro or parsley – finely chopped
¼ t salt or to taste
¼ t cayenne, optional

1. Baked potatoes @ 400°F for 1 hour or until soft to squeeze. Cut in half lengthwise. Scoop out inside, leave ¼-inch thickness near skin. (Save insides for other uses).
2. Sauté onions and garlic until fragrant and brown over medium heat. Add mushrooms and salt, plus 1 t water if needed. Cook briefly with cover on. Keep warm in pan.
3. Combine avocado, tomato and walnuts in a bowl. Add lemon juice, cilantro or parsley, salt, and cayenne if using.
4. To serve: stuff potato halves with mushroom mixtures divided equally among them. Top with avocado mixture.

The Mexi-Potatoes with Baby Bella and Guacamole show case the versatility of one of America's favorite food. This dish provides an abundance of healing nutrients.

For women who are at risk of hormone-dependent breast cancer, the mushrooms have been shown to be a significant source of conjugated linolenic acid (CLA) – a unique type of fatty acid that can bind to aromatase enzymes and lessen the production of estrogen. Since some breast cancer tumors are dependent upon estrogen for growth, this blocking of the aromatase enzymes by the mushrooms' CLA may lower risk of this breast cancer type.

Recent studies have found significant amounts of vitamin B12 in samples of fresh mushrooms. The B12 apparently produced by healthy bacteria growing on the surface of the fresh mushrooms.

Avocados have been shown to inhibit the growth of prostate cancer, destroy oral cancer cells and prevent breast cancer. Avocados contain folate, vitamin E, monounsaturated fats, and glutathione – all are great for your heart, lower risk of stroke, and cancer. Avocados are rich in lutein that protects against macular degeneration and cataracts.

Tomatoes are loaded with lycopene, a vital antioxidant that can flush out the free radicals in the body and fight against cancerous cell formation. Cancers such as prostate, cervical, colon, rectal, stomach, mouth, pharynx and esophagus have all been proven to be staved off by high levels of lycopene.

BREADS AND CRACKERS

Corn Bread
Corn Muffin
Fresh Corn Cornbread
Oat Crackers
No Knead Bread
No Knead Date and Raisin Bread

Corn Bread   yield: 9" X 13" baking pan

3½ c yellow corn meal
3 c whole wheat pastry flour
1/3 c maple syrup powder or other unrefined sugar
2 T baking powder
2 t salt
3½ c soy milk or almond or rice milk
2 c fresh or frozen corn
1 c unsweetened applesauce or 2 peeled apples

1. Preheat oven to 400°F, grease baking pan
2. In a large bowl, combine corn meal, flour, sweetener, baking powder, and salt. Mix well.
3. In Vita-mix, blend corn with part of soymilk until smooth.
4. Add applesauce and remain soymilk to corn-mixture in blender. Process briefly until well mixed.
5. Pour the liquid mixture to flour mixture. Mix well.
6. Pour into prepared baking pan. Bake for 30-35 minutes until tooth pick comes out clean and top golden color.

This cornbread is heavier than those made with eggs and butter. When it is made with fresh sweet corn in season, the taste is delicious. Store the extra cornbread in the refrigerator. Reheat in toaster oven.

Corn contains slow digesting complex carbohydrates and fiber that can control blood sugar levels. However, corn has high glycemic index that needs to be watched by those with diabetes.

Soymilk is made by combining dried soybeans in water, resulting in a similar nutritional content to that of regular cow's milk. However, soymilk contains no trans-fats, no cholesterol; and no synthetic hormones and antibiotics. A serving of soymilk provides more than a third of the USDA's recommended riboflavin, a B vitamin. It acts as an antioxidant, preventing damage to human cells.

A serving of soymilk contains 299 mg calcium, comparable to a glass of cow's milk. It also provides more than half of the vitamin D daily requirement. Vitamin D protects us against cancer, stroke, heart disease, depression, and more. Studies have shown that diets high in soy consumption can reduce the risks of certain types of cancer, as well as menopausal problems.

Corn Muffin

Yield: 6 muffins

1 c frozen corn-thawed or fresh corn
~ ½ –3/4 c non-dairy milk (soy, rice, almond or cashew)
½ t salt
1 c fine cornmeal
1 t baking powder

1. Preheat oven to 350°F. Prepare muffin pans using disposable muffin cups or using non-stick muffin pan.
2. In a blender, blend corn and non-dairy milk until it becomes "corn milk."
3. Add salt and gradually add cornmeal using "pulse" button.
4. Add baking powder and "pulse" briefly. Pour into prepared muffin pan and bake for 25-30 minutes until done by inserting a tooth pick that comes out clean.

You can double the recipe but process the ingredients in two batches, unless you have a powerful blender. With a Vita-mix you can double the recipe which will yield 1 dozen muffins that also will fit an 8" X 8" baking dish or 2 mini-loaf bread pans.

Fresh Corn Cornbread   Yield: 9" X 13" baking pan

1 package (1 T) baking yeast
¾ cup warm water
¾ cup warm soy milk
1/3 c – ½ c agave nectar or maple syrup
3 fresh ears of corn (~3 ½ c fresh corn)
1 c soy milk
1 ¼ c – unbleached all-purpose flour
1 c whole wheat pastry flour
1 ½ – 2 c fine corn meal
1 t salt

1. Dissolve yeast in warm water and warm soy milk (110-115°F). Add sweetener to yeast mixture.
2. Cut corn off the cob. Blend corn and soymilk in blender until smooth. If you prefer some texture, you can set aside ¼ c whole corn kernels.
3. Combine yeast mixture with blended corn in a large bowl.
4. Add flour, corn meal, whole corn kernels (if using) and salt. Mix well.
5. Pour mixture into a greased baking pan. Let rise.
6. Bake at 375°F for 30-35 minutes. (To prevent the top crust get too tough or dried out, bake with cover for 20 minutes, take off cover for the final 10 minutes until edges turn brown and tooth pick comes out clean).

This recipe uses yeast rather than baking powder as the leavening agent. Without eggs and butter, the cornbread is heavier.

Corn has high-quality phyto-nutrition profile comprising of dietary fiber, vitamins, antioxidants, and minerals. Yellow corn has significant levels of flavonoid antioxidants which help to protect us from lung and oral cavity cancers, aging, and inflammation.

Oat Crackers

4 c rolled oats
1 c raw walnuts
4 T date sugar
1 t salt

1. Process the rolled oats to coarsely fine meal in food processor. Put aside in a large bowl.
2. Process the walnuts to finely ground in food processor.
3. Mix ground walnuts, date sugar, and salt with oats.
4. Add ~ 1 cup water (or cashew milk or soymilk) to knead the mixture into dough.
5. Divide dough into two. Roll out dough into thin ~1/4 inch thickness between wax paper. Repeat with other ½ dough.
6. Place on non-stick cookie sheets – score into desired cracker size. Bake at 300°F for 30-35 minutes.

These crackers are chewy. Some may prefer a finer texture. Just process the oats and walnuts to a finer meal will result in a smoother cracker. For a sweeter cracker add more date sugar.

Oats provide a good supply of magnesium, selenium, manganese and phosphorus. They are also a good source of vitamin B1 and fiber. The protein in oats is almost equivalent to the quality of soy protein, and makes it the ideal food for everyone.

While dates contain high amounts of natural sugars, they are actually a low-glycemic index and do not significantly raise blood sugar levels. Dates are loaded with fiber is known to help lower cholesterol and triglycerides which prevent heart disease, stroke and colorectal cancer. Dates are rich in the B vitamins, with vitamin B-6 topping the list. Dates are an excellent source of all the minerals.

No Knead Bread

1½ c whole wheat flour
1 ½ c unbleached all-purpose flour
½ t yeast
1 ½ t salt
1 ½ c water

1. In a glass bowl combine the ingredients. Knead few times in the bowl and shape into a ball. Cover with plastic wrap. Sit at room temperature for 18–24 hours.
2. Dust counter top with flour. Knead the dough 2 to 3 times. Cover with plastic wrap. Let it sit for 2 hours on the counter.
3. Preheat large deep baking pan with lid or a Dutch oven at 450°F for 15 minutes. Place rounded dough into heated baking container. Cover with lid and bake for 30 minutes. Uncover, bake for 10-15 minutes until golden brown. Take lid off and cover with kitchen towel. Let cool, slice and enjoy.

No Knead Date and Raisin Bread

1 c whole wheat flour
2 cup unbleached all-purpose flour
½ t yeast
1 t salt
½ c dates soaked in 1 ¼ c water
¼ c raisins soaked in ¼ cup water, drained. Save the liquid

1. Blend ½ c dates in 1¼ c water and raisin-water in the blender until smooth.
2. In a glass bowl combine the dry ingredients. Knead few times in the bowl and shape into a ball. Cover with plastic wrap. Sit at room temperature for ~15 hours.
3. Dust counter top with flour. Knead the dough few times. Dust flour in the baking pan. Place dough in the baking pan. Cover with plastic wrap. Let it rise for ~1 to 2 hours in the baking pan.
4. Bake in preheat oven at 425°F for ~25-30 minutes with lid on. Uncover and bake ~5 minutes until golden brown. Take lid off and cover with kitchen towel. Let cool, slice and enjoy.

Our daughter in-law Kyle introduced this No Knead Bread. It's simple and quick. Nothing taste better than homemade bread!

DESSERTS

Avocado – Carob Pudding
Carob – Nut Bars
Apple Oat Muffins
Raw Oatmeal Cookies
Almond Butter Carob-Coated-Raisin Cookies
Red Beans and Rice Pudding
Carrot Cake
Hemp - Walnut Clusters
Tapioca Pudding from Sago Palm Pearls
Banana – Cashew Pudding

Avocado – Carob Pudding

3 avocados
3–4 T agave nectar
2 T carob powder
3 T raw creamy almond butter
½ t lemon juice
¼ t cinnamon powder
¼ t nutmeg

1. Put all ingredients in the food processor. Puree until smooth and creamy.
2. Chill in the refrigerator and serve.

The Avocado – Carob Pudding keeps well in the refrigerator for several days. This is a raw dessert full of live enzymes.

Even though avocados are high in fat, they contain monounsaturated fats and cholesterol lowering plant sterols. Monounsaturated fats can actually help you lose belly fat – a known factor in heart disease. Among all nuts, I consider raw almonds as the "king" of nuts. Almonds contain protein, fiber, rich in calcium and vitamins E and folic acid

Carob powder is from pods of a Mediterranean evergreen tree. It is a substitute for cocoa powder but without its fat and caffeine. Carob contains calcium, phosphorus, and iron.

Carob – Nut Bars

4 c raw walnuts – finely ground

1c raw almonds, or cashews or macadamias – finely ground

1 c raw sunflower seeds – finely ground

1 c raw pumpkin (pepitas) seeds – finely ground

4 soft dates – chopped fine and soak in little water

1 c dried shredded unsweetened coconut

½ cup raw carob powder

¼ t salt

1 c raw almond butter at room temperature

1/4 c raw agave nectar or maple syrup

1. In a food processor with S blade, process the walnuts until fine meal-like. But do not over process into "butter." Put in a large bowl.
2. Process the next three ingredients (almonds, sunflower seeds, pumpkin seeds) until finely milled. Add softened dates until well combined. Add to the walnuts.
3. Add coconut, carob powder and salt to the nut-seed mixture. Mix well and set aside.
4. Mix almond butter with agave nectar until well blended. Add to the nut-seed mixture. Combine well.
5. Use gloved-hands mix all ingredients until thoroughly mixed. Sit down and take time to combine the ingredients.
6. Place in a rectangular pan (7" X 11"). Press down and pack firmly using palm of hands or back of spoon.
7. Refrigerate for few hours until hardened or overnight. Cut into squares or bars with a sharp knife. They also freeze well.

The Carob – Nut Bars are indeed nutrition power bars. Walnuts provide essential omega-3 fatty acids, antioxidants, phytosterols, and melatonin creating a powerful cancer-fighting food.

Almonds contain the natural laetrile which has anti-cancer properties. The magnesium helps in reducing the bad LDL cholesterol while increasing the good HDL cholesterol. Almonds help to stabilize the blood sugar levels, benefit those with diabetes.

Sunflower seeds are an exceptional source of vitamin E which has been shown to reduce the risk of colon, bladder, and prostate cancer. Only a quarter of a cup of sunflower seeds can provide you with over 90% of the daily value of vitamin E and over 30% of selenium. Selenium has been shown to induce DNA repair and synthesis in damaged cells.

Pumpkin seeds have phytosterols - compounds that can lower cholesterol and protect against cancers. One half cup of raw pumpkin seeds contain 92% of your daily value of magnesium, a mineral in which most Americans are deficient.

Carob powder is ground from carob pod, free from caffeine, theobromine, and cholesterol. Carob is a rich source of protein, vitamins, minerals, antioxidants, and anti-inflammatory compounds.

Apple Oat Muffins Yield ~24 mini muffins or 10–12 muffins

2 large apples (3 small apples) peeled – finely shredded
2 c rolled oats
½ t salt
½ c dates – chopped, soaked in small amount water and mashed
½ c walnuts

1. Process apples with a shredder disk in the food processor. Place in a large bowl.
2. Process walnuts with the S blade in the food processor until coarsely chopped.
3. Combine the shredded apples with rolled oats, salt, dates and walnuts. If the mixture appears dry, moisten with ~1/4 cup water, adding 1 tablespoon at a time.
4. Pack lightly into muffin pans, round top nicely.
5. Bake at 375° F for 20 minutes or until golden brown.

This recipe is naturally sweet without additional sweetener. Instead of dates, you can use raisins. These mini muffins can be served with breakfast or as a healthy dessert.

Apples, oats and walnuts all combat cancer and protect against heart diseases. Apples are rich in flavonoids and polyphenolics. These compounds help the body protect from deleterious effects of free radicals.

Apples are rich fiber. The peel contains the most of the fiber. Soluble fiber such as pectin actually helps to prevent cholesterol buildup in the lining of blood vessel walls. In addition, the fiber protects the colon mucous membrane from to toxic substances by binding to cancer-causing chemicals inside the colon. Apple contains vitamin C a powerful natural antioxidant which helps the body against infectious agents and scavenges harmful free radicals. Almost half of the vitamin C is just beneath the peel.

Raw Oatmeal Cookies   Yield: 2 dozen 2 ½" X ½" cookies

¾ c raw almonds
3 c rolled oats
1 c medjool dates ((~14 dates)
½ c raisins
2 apples – peeled and cored (~ 1 c apple puree)

1. Place raw almonds in food processor with S blade. Process the almonds to a coarse meal.
2. Add rolled oats and continue process to coarse-fine meal.
3. Gradually add dates to food processor and continue to blend until dough is formed. Put into a large bowl.
4. Add raisins to the dough mixture, blend in well.
5. Puree apples in a blender with a little water (1–2 t).
6. Add to dough mixture and combine well.
7. Form cookies with hand into desired size and thickness (approximately 2 ½" by ½" thick).
8. Place on mesh sheets. Bake in dehydrator at 100°F for 20-24 hours or until the desired crunchiness.

Using the dehydrator, you can "bake" these cookies and yet still retain all the heat sensitive enzymes and vitamins. It is necessary to replenish our enzyme reserves. As one ages, the enzyme reserves tend to deplete quickly.

Apples contain the largest amount of quercetin and ellagic acid, disease-fighting phytochemicals that kill cancer cells. Apples also can protect your heart, correct diarrhea, and cushion the joints.

Almond Butter Carob-Coated-Raisin Cookies

1 (16 oz.) jar raw creamy or chunky almond butter
1 (23 oz.) jar organic unsweetened applesauce
½ c organic raisins – chopped
1 T raw carob powder
½ c to 1 c dates – chopped
2 t cinnamon powder
2 t alcohol free vanilla extract or almond extract
4 c rolled oats

1. Preheat oven to 350°F.
2. In a large bowl mix together almond butter and applesauce until well blended.
3. Shake raisins and carob powder in a bag or a small container with cover until raisins are well coated. Set aside.
4. Add the remaining ingredients and combine well. Stir in carob-coated raisins.
5. Shape dough into desired size balls. Flatten with hand on non-stick baking pan. Bake at 350°F for 30-40 minutes until golden brown. Make approximately 20 large cookies (2 ½") or 40 smaller ones.

In this recipe, instead of using carob chips, I use pure carob powder to coat the raisins to imitate chocolate chips. Most carob chips contain sugar and oil. Again, take time to read the ingredients.

Because the sweetness in this recipe comes from the raisins and dates; you can use more of the dried fruit to suit your taste. Some prefer the larger cookies for its soft "bready" texture; others prefer the crispier smaller cookies.

Almonds provide protective antioxidants against free radical damages and help maintain the integrity of our cells. Almonds contain vitamin E which reduces the risk of cancer and heart disease.

Red Beans and Rice Pudding

3 c cooked or canned red or red kidney beans
3 c cooked sweet brown rice (sticky kind)
4 T unrefined whole cane sugar
½ c – 1 c soy or rice or coconut milk (to desired thickness)
6 soft dates – soak in ½ c water, mash with fork
¾ c raw walnuts – chopped

1. In a large pan, combine cooked beans, cooked rice, sugar and non-dairy milk; simmer on low heat until bubbly and warm. Stir occasionally. If too thick, add little water.
2. Add dates until well combined. Turn off heat.
3. Stir in chopped nuts and serve hot. Or chill in refrigerator for cold pudding.

If you use coconut milk, make sure it does not contain sugar or preservatives. There is a brand of coconut milk without chemicals – AROY-D coconut milk, product of Thailand. Ingredients: coconut-extract and water. Many Asian markets carry it. Trader Joe's coconut milk also does not have any preservatives.

The Red Beans and Rice Pudding can be enjoyed either hot or cold. Save time, you can cook the beans ahead and keep refrigerated. The sticky sweet brown rice can also be cooked ahead. Many Chinese restaurants serve a similar pudding using red and or mung beans and tapioca. The restaurant's pudding contains too much refined sugar. If you prefer a sweeter taste, add more dates or stir in little agave nectar.

Red beans provide nutrients that can protect your heart, stabilize blood sugar, lower cholesterol, and combat cancer. Furthermore, red beans are rich in vitamin B1 (thiamine) which can help improve one's memory, combats depression, fatigue, and lowers Alzheimer's risks. In fact all beans and legumes are chock full of phytochemicals.

Whole grain brown rice contains important B vitamins, minerals, vitamin E, and selenium. The sweet brown rice with its gelatinous property gives nice texture to puddings.

Carrot Cake

2 large carrots – shredded
¼ c organic raisins – soaked in 1/3 c water. Drain. Save the liquid.
5 dates – chopped and soaked in ¼ c water
1 T flax seeds – grind in coffee grinder. (Mix the flax seed meal with 6 T water to use as egg replacer)
½ cup unsweetened applesauce
2 T agave nectar
1 t cinnamon
¼ c walnuts – chopped
~1/3 c Grape-Nut cereal
2 c whole wheat pastry flour
1 t baking powder
1 t baking soda
¼ t salt

1. Preheat oven to 350°F. Shred carrots in food processor using shredder disk. Take out and set aside.
2. Put soaked dates and liquid and raisin water in blender to make a smooth puree.
3. Process applesauce, agave nectar, date puree, cinnamon and flax egg replacer in food processor till well mixed. Add shredded carrots and raisins. Use pause button to combine.
4. In a large mixing bowl, combine pastry flour, baking powder, baking soda and salt. Make a well in center.
5. Add carrot mixture to the dry ingredients. Stir in walnuts and Grape-Nut cereal. Mix thoroughly. Pour into 8" X 8" non-stick baking pan. Bake for 35 – 40 minutes until toothpick inserted in center comes out clean. Cool.

Many versions of carrot cake recipes exist. I have finally developed this one that can be considered a truly healthy one.

Carrot Cake recipes sometimes can be misleading as being "healthy" because it contains carrots. It is said that the molecules in the carrot are closest to human hemoglobin molecules. With its spectrum of nutrients, carrots are indeed beneficial in blood-building and healing. Carrots are particularly important in maintaining healthy epithelial tissues surrounding internal organs. Epithelial tissues are susceptible to cancerous growths.

Walnuts contain antioxidants and anti-inflammatory phytonutrients that can decrease the risk of cancers, and protect against cardiovascular problems, metabolic syndrome and diabetes.

Dates and raisins are full of fiber, vitamins and minerals. Whole wheat flour contains phytochemicals that help to protect against cancer, cardiovascular disease and diabetes.

Hemp -Walnut Clusters   Yield 2 dozen clusters

4 dates – chopped and soaked in ½ c water
½ c raw walnuts
¼ t ground cinnamon
1 "pinch" salt
¼ c raw shelled hemp seeds
1 T raw agave nectar

1. Soak chopped dates in water.
2. Chop walnuts into small pieces. Place in a large bowl.
3. Add cinnamon and salt to walnuts, mix well. Add hemp seeds and combine well.
4. Process soaked dates and agave nectar in blender until smooth. Pour into the nut-seed mixture. Combine.
5. Using spoon and drop individual clusters (size of a large grape or cherry) onto a plate. Place in freezer to set. Enjoy the clusters as a treat or over salad greens. Keep refrigerated.

You can make The Hemp-Walnut Clusters in a jiffy. Make it on a hot summer day, when no cooking is needed. This is a raw recipe; full of goodness and it will enrich your "enzyme bank!"

Some may not be familiar with hemp seeds. Use the hulled hemp seeds. They look like sesame seeds and taste like sunflower seeds. Hemp seeds contain easily digested protein with all the essential amino acids. Just 3 tablespoons provides 11 grams of protein. Hemp seeds also provide a balanced ratio of omega-6 to omega-3 fatty acids. It contains a beneficial gamma linolenic acid (GLA) - important building block of anti-inflammatory hormones. This hormone is important in fat burning for weight loss, helpful for inflammatory conditions, and lowers bad LDL cholesterol.

Walnuts provide antioxidants and anti-inflammatory phytonutrients which can decrease risk of prostate and breast cancer.

Dates are full of fiber, vitamins, and minerals. Dates have been shown to reduce the risk of abdominal cancer.

Tapioca Pudding from Sago Palm Pearls

1 package of sago pearls (use 2 c sago pearls cooked and soaked)
3½ cup water
½ c orange juice
4 T agave nectar or to taste

1. Cook sago palm pearls according to package direction.
2. Put soaked and drained sago pearls in fresh water in a sauce pan over low to medium heat – as it thickens stir to prevent sticking until sago becomes translucent. Turn off heat.
3. Add orange juice and agave nectar. Cool and refrigerate.

Sago palm pearls are used in pudding, fruit soups, smoothies, sides, main dishes, bread, and as a thickening agent. Sago is extracted from the stems of sago palm trees. Sago tastes like tapioca. But tapioca comes from cassava. Sago is low in fat, fiber, and protein. It is low in glycemic index. Sago seems to lower the risk of colon cancer.

Banana – Cashew Pudding

1 c cashew cream* See below
1 ripe banana – cut into chunks
1 T agave nectar
1 t vanilla flavoring
1 T or more water for blending
Pinch salt
½ banana caramelize with 1 T date sugar, optional
Cashew pieces, optional

1. Process the cashew cream, banana chunks, agave, vanilla, salt, and water in a blender until smooth. Add 1 teaspoon water as needed to process it to a pudding-like creaminess.
2. Transfer to serving dessert dishes and chill in the refrigerator.
3. To caramelize the banana slices, coat each slice into the date sugar. Place in a non-stick skillet over medium heat until brown, then carefully turn over to brown other side. To serve, garnish the pudding with caramelized banana slices and scatter few cashews over it.

*Cashew Cream:

1 c raw cashews soak in 4 c hot water or overnight on counter
1/3 c to ½ c cold water

1. Drain soaked cashews and blend in blender with cold water until creamy and smooth.
2. Keep in glass jar for up to one week in the refrigerator. Makes 1 cup Cashew Cream.

The Banana – Cashew Pudding, a simple raw dessert. When the Cashew Cream is made up before hand, it takes only few minutes to prepare this dessert. For variety, you can garnish the pudding with any fruit in season instead of the caramelized banana slices.

MISCELLANEOUS

SAUCES, GRAVY and DIPS
All Purpose Sauce
All Purpose Marinade
Thickened Marinade Sauce
Raw Cashew White Sauce
Creamy White Sauce
Cashew Nut Gravy
Almond and White Bean Dip

Homemade Soy Yogurt

SEEDS and TOPPINGS
Seed Toppings
Seasoned Sesame Seeds
Parmesan Cheese

Homemade Almond Butter

Ben's Spicy Kale Chips – Raw

EGG REPLACER and BINDING AGENT

SAUCES, GRAVY AND DIPS

All Purpose Sauce

1 small onion (1 c) – chopped fine
1/3 c garlic – chopped fine
1 chili pepper – chopped fine
2 T ginger – chopped
Juice of 1 lemon, and lemon peel – chopped
½ c Bragg Liquid Aminos

1. Place 2 c water in frying pan, bring to boil
2. Add onions, continue to simmer until translucent
3. Add garlic, chili pepper and ginger, continue simmer. Add more water if needed.
4. Add lemon juice and peel and liquid aminos. Stir and simmer briefly. Cool and store in the refrigerator.

This All Purpose Sauce can be served over rice, pasta, noodles, potatoes, vegetable salads, vegetables and casseroles. The condiments (onions, garlic, chili peppers, ginger and lemon) contain potent anti-cancer compounds.

All Purpose Marinade

½ cup warm water
1 T unrefined sugar
¼ c Bragg Liquid Aminos
4–6 cloves of garlic – minced
1 chili pepper – minced, optional

1. In a bowl whisk warm water and sugar until dissolved.
2. Add all other ingredients.
3. Marinate the food item for 30 minutes or overnight.

The All Purpose Marinade makes plain unflavored foods tasty. I use it to marinate tofu, gluten, tempeh, mushrooms, seitan, unflavored dehydrated soy products, kelp, and veggies.

Thickened Marinade Sauce

2 T Bragg Liquid Aminos
2 t arrowroot powder (cornstarch)
~1/2 c water

1. Place approximately 2 cups of food item (dehydrated gluten, soy products, tofu, mushrooms etc.) in a large container.
2. Pour marinade over the food, if needed add more water to cover the ingredients. Marinate for one hour or overnight.
3. Sauté over medium heat. Stir and add more water if needed. Cover and cook until done and most liquids are absorbed.

The marinated "meat" can be served alone or combined with other vegetables. I also use this Thickened Marinade as gravy over vegetables, potatoes and noodles.

Raw Cashew White Sauce

½ c raw cashews – soak in ½ cup water
¼ t cumin powder
1 t onion powder
¼ t salt
1 red bell peppers as garnish – chopped

1. Blend all ingredients in blender until smooth.
2. Pour over cooked vegetables. Sprinkle chopped fresh red bell peppers or dried crushed peppers.

This raw recipe seems to dress up any dish in a jiffy. Just pour the Raw Cashew White Sauce over cooked vegetables; garnish with fresh red bell peppers. It adds a new taste to steamed or cooked vegetables. The sauce also makes a nice topping over baked potatoes.

Creamy White Sauce

½ c raw cashews soak in 2 c water
1 t salt
1 t onion powder
1 t garlic powder
2 t arrowroot powder

1. Blend ingredients in blender until smooth.
2. Simmer in small sauce pan until bubbly. Stir. Serve over pasta or cooked vegetables.

Cashew Nut Gravy

1 c water
1 T raw cashews
1 T onion powder
½ t garlic powder
1T arrowroot powder or cornstarch
1T Bragg Liquid Aminos

Place all ingredients in a blender and process until smooth. Pour into a small saucepan and cook over low heat until thickened. Stir frequently, add water if too thick. This versatile gravy can be used over cooked pasta, noodles, potatoes, rice or a main entrée.

Almond and White Bean Dip

¼ c raw almonds
3 cloves of garlic – minced
1 T rosemary leaves – chopped
2 c canned white beans – drained
1 t salt
1/8 t cayenne, optional

1. In a skillet, toast almonds over medium heat for 2–3 minutes. Stir until slightly toasted but not burned. Take out to cool.
2. In the same skillet add 3–4 T water, sauté garlic and rosemary for 1–2 minutes.
3. Process the garlic-rosemary mixture, beans and seasonings in the food processor until smooth. Add toasted almonds and 2–3 T water, process until almonds are finely chopped.

The Almond and White Bean Dip can be used with raw veggies, toasted pita bread, crackers, sandwich or baked chips.

The antioxidants in white beans protect our cells from damages that lead to degenerative diseases. The beans contain molybdenum, a mineral that neutralizes toxins.

Rosemary prevents breast cancer by stimulating liver enzymes that control the estrogen hormone levels in the body. Rosemary is rich in vitamin A known to protect against lung and oral cavity cancers.

Homemade Soy Yogurt   Yield: ~5 cups of soy yogurt

1 container soy yogurt (no refined sugar, no dairy) as starter
1 quart West Soy organic unsweetened soymilk
3 pint-size glass jars with lid

1. In a large stainless steel pot fill half pot with water over medium heat.
2. While heating the water, divide evenly the West Soy milk into 3 jars approximately 3/4 full.
3. Place 2 T of soy yogurt starter into each jar. Stir to mix. Place lids on jars loosely.
4. Place jars into the pot when water temperature reaches to120°F. Turn off heat. Cover pan with lid. Let it sit on stove.

To Test the correct water temperature:

1. Using a cooking thermometer, test the water temperature until it reaches 120°F. Turn off heat.
2. If you do not have a thermometer, use the "finger/hand" test: dip your fingers into the hot water, if you can momentarily leave your fingers in the water before pulling out – that is the correct temperature. Turn off the heat, immediately place the yogurt jars into the water bath and cover the pan with the lid. The pan can just remain on the stove for approximately 4–5 hours. If the temperature of water drops, *momentarily* turn on the stove to low and quickly turn off again.

On sunny hot days, you can move the pan with the hot water outdoors and let the solar energy heat the pan for 4 to 5 hours. The yogurt will be softly-firm. Store the yogurt in the refrigerator for 2 weeks. Save one jar as a starter for the next batch. If you live in an area where the sun light is quite intense for 4 hours, then you can just put the yogurt jars on a table outdoors without the water bath. Generally, the yogurt will be done in 3 hours.

I want to give credit to my sister who developed the "finger/hand" testing method which appears to be more "scientific" than my cooking thermometer!

SEEDS AND TOPPINGS

Seed Toppings

Use equal amounts of the following:
Sesame seeds, raw
Flax seeds, raw
Pumpkin seeds, raw
Sunflower seeds, raw

1. In a seed or "coffee" grinder, grind sesame seeds to a fine powder. Continue grind the next seeds.
2. Place all ground seeds in a large bowl and mix well. Store in a glass jar and keep in the refrigerator. Use within one week.

The ground seeds can be sprinkled on any food. This recipe provides excellent sources of essential amino acids, fatty acids, minerals; rich in vitamin E, fiber and live enzymes.

Just ½ c of sesame seeds contains three times more calcium than ½ c of milk. Sesame seeds also provide substances that prevent high blood pressure and protect the liver against oxidative damage.

Flax seeds contain more lignans (antioxidants) than any other plant foods that provide protection against cancers, particularly breast cancer by blocking enzymes that are involved in hormone metabolism, and interfering the growth and spread of tumor.

Pumpkin seeds (pepitas) are loaded with compounds that help combat cancer by killing various types of cancer cells as breast cancer and prostate cancer.

Sunflower seeds are rich in vitamin E which helps to protect cells against free radical damages. One ounce of sunflower seeds provides 35 percent of a person's daily need of vitamin E. Sunflower seeds contain copper that is excellent for healthy skin and hair. Just one ounce of sunflower seeds provides more than 50 percent of the recommended daily intake for copper.

Seasoned Sesame Seeds

¼ c sesame seeds
1 t garlic powder
½ t salt
¼ t oregano or thyme powder (2 t dried herbs)

1. Toast sesame seeds in toaster oven till golden brown.
2. Combine with seasonings. When cool, store in a tight jar. If you have a salt-shaker with large holes, you can store the seasoned sesame seeds in it. Shake on dips, salads, rice, pasta and other dishes.

Parmesan Cheese

¼ c sesame seeds
2 t onion powder
½ c nutritional yeast
½ t salt

1. Toast sesame seeds lightly in 350°F oven or toaster oven.
2. Grind toasted seeds. Combine with remaining ingredients.

This makes a nice topping for spaghetti, pasta or salads.

Homemade Almond Butter – *Using Champion Juicer*:

1 c whole raw almonds with skin – keep in freezer over night

1. Using a Champion Juicer with a blank plate, while running, drop a handful of frozen almonds into the chute. Push through slowly with a plunger. The frozen almonds will come out as almond butter.
2. Keep it in a glass jar in the refrigerator. One cup raw almonds yield approximately 1 cup almond butter.

Using Vita-Mix Dry Container:

2 c raw almonds – soaked overnight and drained

1. Place soaked and drained almonds into the dry container in the Vita-Mix. Blend on high until smooth and creamy, using the plunger to push it down.
2. Store it in glass jar in the refrigerator.

Raw almonds are excellent sources of the antioxidant selenium; minerals including calcium, phosphorus, magnesium; vitamin E, protein and fiber. Almonds contain good monounsaturated fat which helps lower cholesterol and reduce heart disease and cancer; and increase longevity.

Ben's Spicy Kale Chips – Raw

1 package (10 oz.) kale or 1 bunch fresh kale – (center hard stem removed and cut leaves to chip size)
2 sheets of raw nori seaweed
1 T olive oil
1 T Bragg Liquid Aminos
1 T nutritional yeast
1 T dehydrated minced onions
½ t salt to taste
2–3 shakes of cayenne, optional
2–3 shakes of dried crushed red peppers, optional

1. Place all ingredients in a large container. Massage well.
2. Place on 4 trays lined with teflex in dehydrator @ 118°F for 2 hours or until desired crispiness.

Nori seaweeds are paper thin sheets of dried seaweed. They contain protein, dietary fiber, vitamins and minerals.

Just one cup kale provides 1,327 percent of daily Vitamin K. This vitamin protects against various cancers and Alzheimer's disease. Kale furnishes 192 percent of vitamin A and 89 percent of vitamin C. Per calorie, kale has more calcium than milk, and more iron than beef. Kale is rich with fiber and sulfur.

EGG REPLACER and BINDING AGENT:

Stir 1 T ground hemp seeds into 3 T water for each egg.
Stir 1 T flaxseed meal into 3 T water or juice per egg.
Grind 1 T flax seeds into powder. Stir into 6 T water for two eggs.
Soak 1 T whole flax seeds. Cover with water, let set. The liquid becomes "egg white like gel".

APPENDIX

Health Educational Institutes and Wellness Centers in the U.S. and Asia:

Here is a partial list of places one can go to learn how to take care of most major diseases through diet and lifestyle changes. They are educational centers, not treatment centers.

Gerson Institute
P. O. Box 161358
San Diego, CA 92176
Office:
3844 Adams Ave
San Diego, CA 92116
1-888-443-7766 US and Canada
1-800-838-2256 US only
1-619-685-5353 Best for local and international callers

Hallelujah Acres
P. O. Box 2388
900 S. Post Road
Shelby, NC 28152
1-800-915-9355
www.hacres.com

Hartland Institute of Health and Education
444 Hartland Oak Drive
Rapidan, VA 22733
540-672-3100
E-mail: info@hartland.edu

Hippocrates Health Institute
1443 Palmdale Court
West Palm Beach, FL 33411
561-471-9976
HippocratesInst.org

Living Foods Institute
1700 Commerce Dr NW Suite 100 or
1530 Dekalb Ave NE Suite E
Atlanta, GA 30318
1-800-844-9876
404-524-4488
Livingfoodsinstitute.com

John A. McDougall, M.D.
Dr. McDougall's Health and Medical Center
P. O. Box 14039
Santa Rosa, CA 95402
1-800-941-7111
707-538-8609
www.drmcdougall.com

Optimum Health Institute
6970 Central Avenue
Lemon Grove, CA 91945-2198
1-800-993-4325
Tel 619-464-3346
www.optimumhealth.org

Optimum Health Institute
265 Cedar Lane
Cedar Creek, TX 78612
1-800-993-4325
512-303-4817
www.optimumhealth.org

Weimar Center of Health & Education
20601 W. Paoli Lane
Weimar, CA 95736
1-800-525-9192
www.NEWSTART.com

Wildwood Lifestyle Center and Hospital
435 Lifestyle Lane
Wildwood, GA 30757
1-800-634-9355
706-820-1493
www.wildwoodhealth.org/lifestyle

Uchee Pines Institute
30 Uchee Pines Road
Seale, AL 36875-5715
334-855-4781
Ucheepines.com

Aenon Health Care
Lot 961, Jalan Batu Belang-Keru
Mukim Tampin Tengah
Daerah Tampin
73000 Negeri Sembilan
Malaysia
011-(6)012-712-6960
Email@aenon.org.my

References

Introduction

1. American Cancer Society: Estimated new cancer cases and death by sex for all sites, U.S., 2010.
2. National Cancer Institute: Comprehensive cancer incidence and mortality report. www.gov/newscenter, 2011.
3. American Cancer Society: Estimated breast cancer mortality, incidence, and I/M ratios, USA. 2011.
4. www.gits4u.com/health/cancer.htm
5. www.inctr.org/about-inctr/cancer-in-developing-countries
6. healthland.time.com/2014/02/03/cancer-cases
7. Brayand F, and Moller B: Predicting the future burden of cancer. Nat. Rev. Cancer 63-74, 2006. Doi:10.1038/ncr1781.
8. realtruth.org/articles/090203-005-**health**.html
9. http://www.answerstohealthcare.com/articles/american-Healthcare
10. Barnard N: The Cancer Project Report. August 26, 2011.
11. American Institute for Cancer Research/World Cancer Research Fund policy report: Lifestyle Changes Vital for Preventing Cancer. http://www.aicr.org/site/DocServer/UICCprWCD2011.
12. Carmona RH: The Future of Health Care – The Role of Preventive and Integrative Medicine. Loma Linda University 80th Annual Postgraduate Convention. March, 2012
13. Ornish D: Dr. Dean Ornish's Program for Reversing Heart Disease. Random House, Inc., 1990.
14. Esselstyn CB Jr: Prevent and Reverse Heart Disease. Penguin Group (USA) Inc., 2007.
15. Barnard ND: Dr. Neal Barnard's Program for Reversing Diabetes. Rodale, Inc., 2007.
16. Campbell C T, Campbell II TM: The China Study. BenBella Books, Dallas, TX, 2005.
17. McDougall JA: The McDougall Program. Penguin Group (USA) Inc., 1990.

Chapter 1 — Why This Book?

1. Lau BHS, Woolley JL, Marsh CL, Barker GR, Koobs DH, and Torrey RR: Superiority of intralesional immunotherapy with *Corynebacterium parvum* and *Allium sativum* in control of murine transitional cell carcinoma. *Journal of Urology* 136:701-705. 1986.

2. Marsh CL, Torrey RR, Woolley JL, Barker GR, Lau BHS: Superiority of intravesical immunotherapy with *Corynebacterium parvum* and *Allium sativum* in control of bladder tumor. *Journal of Urology* 137:359-362, 1987.

3. Woolley JL, Lau BHS, Ruckle HC, Torrey RR: Phagocytic and natural killer cytotoxic responses of murine transitional cell carcinoma to postsurgical immunochemotherapy. *Journal of Urology* 140:660-663, 1988.

4. Rittenhouse JR, Lui PD, Lau BHS: Chinese medicinal herbs reverse macrophage suppression induced by urological tumors. *Journal of Urology* 146:486-490, 1991.

5. Lau BHS, Ruckle HC, Botolazzo T, Lui PD: Chinese medicinal herbs inhibit growth of murine renal cell carcinoma. Cancer Biotherapy 9:153-161, 1994.

6. Lau BHS, Yamasaki T, Gridley DS: Garlic Compounds modulate macrophage and T-lymphocyte functions. *Molecular Biotherapy* 3:103-107, 1991.

7. Folkman J, Merler E, Abernathy C, Williams G: Isolation of tumor factor responsible for angiogenesis. *Journal of Experimental Medicine* 133:275-288, 1971.

8. Dulak J: Nutraceuticals as anti-angiogenesis agents: Hope and reality. *Journal of Physiology & Pharmacology* 56 (suppl. 1):51-60, 2005.

Chapter 2 — Beginnings of Cancer Research

1. Bergquist LM, Lau BH, Winter CE: Mycoplasma-associated immunosuppression: effect of hemagglutin response to common antigens in rabbits. *Infection and Immunity* 9:410-415, 1974.

2. Slater JM, Ngo E, Lau BHS: Effect of therapeutic irradiation on the immune responses. *American Journal of Roentgenology* 26:313-320, 1976.

3. Wong DS, Masek TD, Slater JM, Lau BHS: Effect of low dose total body irradiation on the in vivo destruction of Friend virus-induced leukemia. *International Journal of Radiation Oncology* 2:168, 1977.

4. Cremer NE: In Virus Tumorigenesis and Immunogenesis (Eds.WS Ceglowski and H Friedman; Academic Press, New York), p. 239, 1973.

5. Friedman H, Ceglowsky WS: in Progress in Immunology (Ed. B Amos; Academic Press, New York), p.815, 1971.

6. Law LW, Dunn TB, Boyle PJ, Miller JH: Observations on the effect of a folic-acid antagonist on transplantable lymphoid leukemia in mice. *Journal of Natioanl Cancer Institute* 10:179-192, 1949.

7. Johnson JA, Lau BHS, Nutter RL, Slater JM, Winter CE: Effect of L1210 leukemia on the susceptibility of mice to *Candida albicans* infections. *Infection and Immunity* 19:146-151, 1978.

8. Lau BHS, Masek TD, Chu WT, Slater JM: Antiinflammatory reaction associated with murine L1210 leukemia. *Experientia* 32:1598-1600, 1976.

9. Gridley DS, Lau BHS, Tosk JM: Phagocytic cell chemiluminescence using different zymosan preparations. *Journal of Clinical Laboratory Analysis* 5:101-105, 1991.

10. Gridley DS, Prabhu MR, Lau BHS, Kettering JD: Modulation of lymphoproliferation and oxidative burst by herpes-transformed tumors. *Molecular Biotherapy* 3:88-94, 1991.

11. Lau BHS, Yamasaki T, Gridley DS: Garlic Compounds modulate macrophage and T-lymphocyte functions. *Molecular Biotherapy* 3:103-107, 1991.

12. Adetumbi MA, Lau BHS: *Allium sativum* (garlic) - a natural antibiotic. *Medical Hypothesis* 12:227-237, 1983.

13. Adetumbi MA, Lau BHS: Inhibition of in vitro germination and spherulation of *Coccidioides immitis* by *Allium sativum*. *Current Microbiology* 13:73-76, 1986.

14. Adetumbi MA, Javor GT, Lau BHS: *Allium sativum* (garlic) inhibits lipid synthesis by *Candida albicans*. *Antimicrobial Agents and Chemotherapy* 30:499-501, 1986.

15. Lau BHS: Garlic for disease prevention. *Journal of Health and Healing* 13:3-6, 1990.

16. Lau BHS, Tadi PP, Tosk JM: *Allium sativum* (garlic) and cancer prevention. *Nutrition Research* 10:937-948, 1990.

17. Tosk J, Lau BHS, Myers, RC, Torrey R: Selenium-induced enhancement of hematoporphyrin derivative phototoxicity in murine bladder tumor cells. *Biochem Biophys Res Comm* 104:1086-1092, 1986.

18. Lau BHS, Wang-Cheng RM, Tosk J: Tumor-specific T-lymphocytes cytotoxicity enhanced by low dose of C. parvum. *Journal of Leukocyte Biology* 41:407-411, 1987.

19. Lau BHS, Marsh CL, Barker GR, Woolley JL, Torrey RR: Effects of biological response modifiers on murine bladder tumor. *Nat Immun Cell Growth Regul* 4:260, 1985.

20. Mei X, Wang ML, Xu HX, Pan XP, Gao CY, Han N, Fu MY: Garlic and gastric cancer. *Acta Nutr Sinica* 4:53-67, 1982.

21. Pan XY: Comparison of the cytotoxic effect of fresh garlic, diallyl trisulfide, 5-fluorouracil, mitomycin C and cis-DDP on two lines of gastric cancer cells. *Chung-Hua Chung Liu Tsa Chih* 7:103-122, 1985.

22. Wargovich MJ, Goldberg MT: Diallyl sulfide: a naturally occurring thioether that inhibits carcinogen-induced nuclear damage to colon epithelial cells in vitro. *Mutation Research* 143:127, 1985.

23. Wargovich MJ: Diallyl sulfide, a flavor component of garlic (Allium sativa), inhibits dimethylhydrazine-induced colon cancer. *Carcinogenesis* 8:487, 1987.

24. Belman S: Onion and garlic oils inhibit tumor promotion. *Carcinogenesis* 4:1063, 1983.

25. Sparnins VL, Mott AW, Barany G, Wattenberg of LW: Effects of allyl methyl trisulfide on glutathione S transferase activity and benzopyrene-induced neoplasia in the mouse. *Nutr Cancer* 8:211, 1986.

26. Servan-Schreiber D: Anticancer – a new way of life. Anticancer Action insert, pages 9-11. Published by Penguin Group, New York, New York. 2009.

27. Lau BHS, Lau EW: Edible plant extracts modulate macrophage activity and bacterial mutagenesis. *International Clinical Nutrition Review* 12:147-155, 1992.

28. Lau EW: A powerhouse of nutrients. *Explore* 4:3-5, 1993.

29. Lau BHS, Lau EW: Kyo-green improves sexual dysfunction in men and women. *Medical Science Monitor* 9:112-118, 2003.

30. Lau BHS, Woolley JL, Marsh CL, Barker GR, Koobs DH, and Torrey RR: Superiority of intralesional immunotherapy with *Corynebacterium parvum* and *Allium sativum* in control of murine transitional cell carcinoma. *Journal of Urology* 136:701-705, 1986.

31. Marsh CL, Torrey RR, Woolley JL, Barker GR, Lau BHS: Superiority of intravesical immunotherapy with C. parvum and Allium sativum in control of bladder tumor. *Journal of Urology* 137:359-362, 1987.

32. Woolley JL, Lau BHS, Ruckle HC, Torrey RR: Phagocytic and natural killer cytotoxic responses of murine transitional cell carcinoma to postsurgical immuno-chemo-therapy. *Journal of Urology* 140:660-663, 1988.

33. Wan CP, Park CS, Lau BHS: A rapid and simple micro-fluorometric phagocytosis assay. *Journal of Immunological Methods* 162:1-7, 1993.

34. Li L, Lau BHS: A simplified in vitro model of oxidant injury using vascular endothelial cells. *In Vitro Cell Dev Biol* 29A:531-536, 1993.

35. Tadi PP, Teel RW, Lau BHS: Anticandidal and anticarcinogenic potentials of garlic. *International Clinical Nutritional Review* 10:423-429, 1990.

36. Tadi PP, Teel RW, Lau BHS: Organosulfur compounds of garlic modulate mutagenesis, metabolism and DNA binding of aflatoxin B1. *Nutrition and Cancer* 15:87-95, 1991.

37. Tadi PP, Lau BHS, Teel RW, Herrmann CE: Binding of aflatoxin B1 to DNA inhibited by ajoene and diallyl sulfide. *Anticancer Research* 11:450-454, 1991.

38. Uppala PT, Dissmore T, Lau BH, Andacht T, Rajaram S: Selective inhibition of cell proliferation by lycopene in MCF-7 breast cancer cells in vitro: a proteomic analysis. *Phytotherapy Research* 27:595-601, 2013.

39. Campbell TC, Campbell II TM: The China Study. Benbella Books, Dallas, TX, 2005.

40. Wigley C: Chemical carcinogenesis and precancer. In Introduction to the Cellular and Molecular Biology of Cancer. L.M. Franks and N. Teich, editors. P 131, 1986.

41. Adams GE: Radiation carcinogenesis. In Introduction to the Cellular and Molecular Biology of Cancer. L.M. Franks and N. Teich, editors. P 154, 1986.

42. Grisebach H, Ebel J: Phytoallexins, chemical defense substances of higher plants? *Angew Chem Int Ed Engl* 17:635-647, 1978.

43. Yamasaki T, Teel RW, Lau BHS: Effect of allixin, a phytoalexin produced by garlic, on mutagenesis, DNA binding, and metabolism of aflatoxin B1. *Cancer Letters* 59:89-94, 1991.

44. Wong BYY, Lau BHS, Teel RW: Chinese medicinal herbs modulate mutagenesis, DNA binding and metabolism of Benzo[a]pyrene. *Phytotherapy Research* 6:10-14, 1991.

45. Wong BYY, Lau BHS, Teel RW: Chinese medicinal herbs modulate mutagenesis, DNA binding and metabolism of benzo[a]pyrene 7,8-dihydrodiol and benzo[a] pyrene 7,8-dihydrodiol-9,10-epoxide. *Cancer Letters* 62:123-131, 1992.

46. Wong BYY, Lau BHS, Tadi PP, Teel RW: Chinese medicinal herbs modulate mutagenesis, DNA binding and metabolism of aflatoxin B1. *Mutation Research* 279:209-216, 1992.

47. Wong BYY, Lau BHS, Yamasaki T, Teel RW: Metabolism of cytochrome P-450IA1-mediated mutagenesis, DNA binding and metabolism of benzo[a] pyrene by Chinese medicinal herbs. *Cancer Letters* 68:75-82, 1993.

48. Wong BYY, Lau BHS, Yamasaki T, Teel RW: Inhibition of dexamethasone-induced cytochrome P450-mediated mutagenecity and metabolism of aflatoxin B1 by Chinese medicinal herbs. *European Journal of Cancer Prevention* 2:351-356, 1993.

49. Wong BYY, Lau BHS, Jia TY, Wan CP: Oldenlandia diffusa and Scutellaria barbata augment macrophage oxidative burst and inhibit tumor growth. *Cancer Biotherapy* 11:51-56, 1996.

50. Wong BYY, Wong HHL: An evicence-based perspective of Scutellaria barbata (Skullcap) for cancer patients. In Evidence-based Anticancer Materia Medica, William CS Cho, editor. Springer, publishers, pages 155-177, 2011.

51. Rittenhouse JR, Lui PD, Lau BHS: Chinese medicinal herbs reverse macrophage suppression induced by urological tumors. *Journal of Urology* 146:486-490, 1991.

52. Lau BHS, Ruckle HC, Botolazzo T, Lui PD: Chinese medicinal herbs inhibit growth of murine renal cell carcinoma. *Cancer Biotherapy* 9:153-161, 1994.

53. Lau BHS, Ong P, Tosk J: Macrophage Chemiluminescence Modulated by Chinese Medicinal Herbs *Astragalus membranaceus* and *Ligustrum lucidum*. *Phytotherapy Research* 3:148-153, 1989.

54. Wang Y, Qian JJ, Hadley HR, Lau BHS: Phytochemicals potentiate IL-2 generated LAK cell cytotoxicity against murine renal cell carcinoma. *Molecular Biotherapy* 4:143-146, 1992.

Chapter 3—More Basic Nutritional Research

1. American Cancer Society: Ovarian Cancer. http:/ www.cancer.org 2000.

2. National Ovarian Cancer Collation: Symptoms of ovarian cancer. 2001.

3. Buz'Zard AR, Lau BHS: Selective toxicity of Pycnogenol˚ for malignant ovarian germ cells in vitro. *International Journal of Cancer Prevention* 1:207-212, 2004.

4. Buz'Zard AR, Lau BHS: Pycnogenol reduces talc-induced neoplastic transformation in human ovarian cell cultures. *Phytotherapy Research* 21:579-586, 2007.
5. Michael Anderson Documentary Film: Healing Cancer From Inside Out. 2008.

Chapter 4 —Adventist Health Study

1. Lau B: The Adventist advantage—a closer look. *Spectrum* 35(4):59-63, 2007.
2. Fraser GE, Shavilk DJ: Ten years of life: Is it a matter of choice? *Archives of Internal Medicine* 161:1645-1652, 2001.
3. Mills PK, Beeson WL, Phillips RL, Fraser GE: Cancer incidence among California Seventh-day Adventists, 1976-1982. *American Journal of Clinical Nutrition* 59 (suppl.):1136S-1142S, 1994.
4. Fraser GE: Association between diet and cancer, ischemic heart disease, and all-cause mortality in non-Hispanic white California Seventh-day Adventists. *American Journal of Clinical Nutrition* 70 (suppl.):532S-538S, 1999.
5. Campbell TC, Campbell II TM: The China Study. Benbella Books, Dallas, Texas. 2005.
6. Chan JM, Giovannucci EL: Dairy products, calcium, and vitamin D and risk of prostate cancer. *Epidemiologic Reviews* 23:87-92, 2001.
7. Park S, Murphy SP, Wilkens LR: Calcium, vitamin D, and dairy product intake and prostate cancer risk—the multi-ethnic cohort study. *American Journal of Epidemiology* 166:1259-1269, 2007.
8. Park Y, Mitrou PN, Kipnis V: Calcium, dairy foods, and risk of incident and fatal prostate cancer risk: NIH-AARP diet and health study. *American Journal of Epidemiology* 166:1270-1279, 2007.
9. Kiani F, Knutsen S, Singh P, Ursin G, Fraser G: Dietary risk factors for ovarian cancer: the Adventist health study (United States). *Cancer Causes Control* 17 (2):137-146, 2006.
10. Larsson SC, Orsinin N, Wolk A: Milk, milk products and lactose intake and ovarian cancer risk: a meta-analysis of epidemiological studies. *International Journal of Cancer* 118:431-441, 2006.
11. Cramer DW, Xu H, Sahi T: Adult hypolactasia, milk consumption and age specific fertility. *American Journal of Epidemiology* 139:282-289, 1994.
12. Ornish D, Weidner G, Fair WR: Intensive lifestyle changes may affect the progression of prostate cancer. *Journal of Urology* 74:1065-1069, 2005.
13. Barnard N: The Cancer Project Report. August 26, 2011.

Chapter 5 — Cancer Immunology Made Simple

1. Male D: Introduction to the, Immune System. In *Immunology*, 6th edition, Mosby, Times Mirror International Publishers Ltd. Pp. 1-12, 2001.

2. Rook GAW: Immunity to Bacteria and Fungi. In *Immunology*, 6th edition, Mosby, Times Mirror International Publishers Ltd. Pp. 245-258, 2001.

3. Trapani JA, Smyth MJ: Functional significance of the perforin/granzyme cell death pathway. *Nature Reviews Immunology* 2:735-747, 2005.

4. Voskoboinik I, Trapani JA: Addressing the mystery of perforin function. *Immunology and Cell Biology* 84:66-71, 2006.

5. Nash T: Immunity to Viruses. In *Immunology*, 6th edition, Mosby, Times Mirror International Publishers Ltd. Pp.235-243, 2001.

6. Lau B: Fat Cat Fights the Immune System. In *Energized —1998 Devotional*. Review & Herald Publishing Association, Hagerstown, MD. P. 103, 1998.

7. Lau B: Sweet and Weak. In *Energized —1998 Devotional*. Review & Herald Publishing Association, Hagerstown, MD. P. 166, 1998.

8. Nixon DW: Nutrition and cancer: American Cancer Society guidelines, programs, and initiatives. *CA-A Cancer Journal for Clinicians* 40:71-76, 1990.

9. Butrum RR, Clifford CK, Lanza E: NCI dietary guidelines: Rationale. *American Journal of Nutrition*. 48:888-895, 1988.

10. Chajes V: Association between serum trans-monounsaturated fatty acids and breast cancer risk in E3N-EPIC study. *American Journal of Epidemiology* 167:1312-1320, 2008.

11. Sanchez A, Reeser JL, Lau BHS: Role of sugars in human neutrophilic phagocytosis. *American Journal of Clinical Nutrition* 26:1180-1184, 1973.

12. Jee SH, Ohrr H, Sull JW: Fasting serum glucose level and cancer risk in Korean men and women. *JAMA* 293:194-202, 2005.

13. Ader R, Felton DL, Cohen N: Psychoneuroimmunology, 2nd edition. Academic Press, New York, 1991.

14. Kiecolt-Glaser JK, Glaser R, Strain JC: modulation of cellular immunity in medical students. *Journal of Behavioral Medicine* 9:5-21, 1986.

15. Palmblad J, Petrini B, Wasserman J, Akerstedt T: Lymphocyte and granulocyte reactions during sleep deprivation. *Psychosomatic Medicine* 41:273-278, 1979.

16. Schleifer SJ, Keller SE, Camerino M, Thornton JC, Stein M: Suppression of lemphocyte stimulation following a bereavement. *JAMA* 250:374-382, 1983.

17. Yahya MD, Watson RR: Immunomodulation by morphine and marijuana. *Life Sciences* 41:2503-2510, 1987.

18. Chao CC, Molitor TW, Gekker G, Murtnugh MP, Peterson PK: Cocaine mediated suppression of superoxide production by human peripheral blood mononuclear cells. *Journal of Pharmacology and Experimental Therapeutics* 256:255-258, 1991.

19. Melamid I, Kark JD, Spirer Z: Coffee and the immune system. *International Journal of Immunopharmacology* 12:129-134, 1990.

20. Szabo G: Consequences of alcohol consumption on host defence. *Alcohol* 34:830-841, 1999.

21. Watson RR: Ethanol, Immunomodulation and Cancer. *Progress in Food and Nutrition Science* 12: 189-209, 1988.

22. Mutchbik MG, Lee HH: Impaired Lymphocyte Response to Mitogen in Alcoholic Patients, *Alcoholism, Clinical and Experimental Research* 12: 155-158, 1988.

23. Glassman AB, Bennett CE, Randall CL: Effects of Ethyl Alcohol on Human Peripheral Lymphocytes. *Archives of Pathology and Laboratory Medicine* 109: 540-542, 1985.

24. Johnson S, Knight R, Marmer DJ, Steele RW: Immune Deficiency in Fetal Alcohol Syndrome. *Pediatric Research* 15:908-911, 1981.

25. Brooks GF, Butel JS, Morse SA: Jawetz, Melnick, & Adelberg's Medical Microbiology, 21th edition, page 212. Appleton & Lange, 1998.

26. Zenebe W, Pechanova O: Effects of Red Wine Polyphenolic Compounds on the Cardiovascular System. *Bratisl Lek Listy* 103:159-165, 2002.

27. Huxley RR, Neil HA: The Relation between Dietary Flavonol Intake and Coronary Heart Disease Mortality: A Meta-analysis of Prospective Cohort Studies. *European Journal of Clinical Nutrition* 57:904-908, 2003.

28. Mukamal KJ, Conigrave KM, Mittleman MA, Camargo CA Jr, Stampfer MJ, Willett WC, Rimm EB: Roles of Drinking Pattern and Type of Alcohol Consumed in Coronary Heart Disease in Men. *New England Journal of Medicine* 348:109-118, 2003.

29. Fernandez-Jarne E, Martinez-Losa E, Serrano-Martinez M, Prado-Santamaria M, Brugarolas-Brufau C, Martinez-Gonzalez MA: Type of Alcoholic Beverage and First Acute Myocardial Infarction: A Case-controlled Study in a Mediterranean Country. *Clinical Cardiology* 26:313-318, 2003.

30. Suh I, Shaten BJ, Cutler JA, Kuller L: Alcohol Use and Mortality from Coronary Heart Disease: the Role of High-density lipoportein cholesterol. The Multiple Risk Factor Intervention Trial Research Group. *Annals of Internal Medicine* 116:881-887, 1992.

31. Vogel, R.A.: Alcohol, Heart Disease, and Mortality: A Review. *Review of Cardiovascular Medicine* 3:7-13, 2002.

32. Johnson, J.D., Houchens, D.P., Kluwe, W.M., Craig, D.K., Fisher, G.L.: Effects of Mainstream and Environmental Tobacco Smoke on the Immune System in Animals and Humans: A Review. *Critical Reviews in Toxicology* 20:369-395, 1990.

33. Mili, F., Flanders, W.D., Boring, J.R., Annest, J.L., Destefano, F. The Asosciations of Race, Cigarette Smoking, and Smoking Cessation to Measures

of the Immune system in Middle-aged Men. *Clinical Immunology and Immunopathology* 59:187-200, 1991.

34. Moszczynski, P., Slowinski, S., Lisiewicz, J.: Effect of Tobacco Smoking on Selected Immunologic Indices. *Folia Haematologica* (Leipz):305-310, 1989.

35. Magnusson, C.G.: Maternal Smoking Influences Cord Serum IgE and IgD Levels and Increases the Risk for Subsequent Infant Allergy. *Journal of Allergy and Clinical Immunology* 78:898-904, 1986.

Chapter 6 — Healing Cancer from Inside Out

1. Cairns J: The treatment of diseases and the war against cancer. *Scientific American* 253(5):51-59, 1985.

2. Abel U: Chemotherapy of advanced epithelial cancer: a critical survey. Hippokrates Verlag Stuttgart 1990.

3. Morgan G, Ward R, Barton M: The contribution of cytotoxic chemotherapy to five-year survival in adult malignancies. *Clinical Oncology* 16:549-560, 2004.

4. Gofman JW: Preventing breast cancer: The X-ray and health project. www.x-rayandhealth.org.

5. Geng Z, Rong Y, Lau BHS: S-allyl cysteine inhibits activation of nuclear factor kappa B in human T cells. *Free Radical Biology & Medicine* 23:345-350, 1997.

6. Campbell TC, Campbell II TM: The China Study. Benbella Books, Dallas, Texas. 2005.

Chapter 7 —Observational Research

1. Slater JM, Ngo E, Lau BHS: Effect of therapeutic irradiation on the immune responses. *American Journal of Roentg* 26:313-320, 1976.

2. Sun Y, Campisi J, Hipano C: Treatment-induced damage to the tumor microenvironment promotes prostate cancer therapy resistance through WNT16B. *Natural Medicine* 10:1038, 2012.

3. Binzel PE: Alive and Well—A doctor's experience with nutrition in the treatment of cancer patients. American Media Publisher, California, 1994.

4. Malkmus GH: Why Christians Get Sick. Hallelujah Acres Publishing, Tennessee, 1989.

Chapter 8 –Toxic Environment

1. Campbell TC, Campbell II TM: The China Study. BenBella Books, Dallas, TX, 2005.

2. Releases of toxic chemicals increased by 8 percent in 2011. Chemical Regulation Reporter January 18, 2013. www2.epa.gov/toxic-release-inventory-tri-protram/tri

3. Organophosphate. En.wikipedia.org/wiki/organophosphate

4. Peattie C: How do chemicals in the environment mimic estrogen? May 22, 2009. www.chem.duke.edu/~jds/cruise-chem/pest/estmim.html

5. http://www.ewg.org/environment.

6. "Corporate Crime," Subcommittee on Crime, U.S. House of Representatives. P.25-28, May 1980.

7. Landrigan PJ, Goldman LR: Children's Vulnerability to Toxic Chemicals: A Challenge and Opportunity to Strengthen Health and Environmental Policy. Publicado em maio 9, 2011 por HC. www.ecodebate.com. br/2011/05/09.

8. Bis(2-ethylhexyl)Phthalate(DEHP). www.epa.gov/ttn/atw/hlthef/eth-phth.html

9. Centers for Disease Control, Third National Report on Human Exposure to Environmental Chemicals. Atlanta: Centers for Disease Control and Prevention. 2005.

10. Silva MJ, Barr DB, Reidy JA, Malek NA, Hodge CC, Caudill SP, Brock JW, Needham LL, Calafat AM: Urinary levels of seven phthalate metabolites in the U.S. population from the National Health and Nutrition Examination Survey (NHANES) 1999-2000. Environ Health Perspective 112(3):331-8, 2004.

11. Taylor R, "Cattle Deaths stir Pesticide Debate," Los Angeles Times Nov 5, 1979.

12. Effects, Uses, Control and Research of Agricultural Pesticides," A Report by the Surveys and Investigations Staff, USDA; Presented at Hearings before a Subcommittee on Appropriations, 89th Congress, first session, House of Representatives, Department of Agricultural Appropriations, part 1, p.174.

13. "Basic Information about Polychlorinated Biphenyls (PCBs) in Drinking Water." United States Environmental Protection Agency. Water.epa.gov/.../polychlorinated-biphenyls.cfm

14. Food and Agriculture Organization of the United Nations (FAO), FAOSTAT on-line statistical service. http://apps.fao.org

15. Factory Farms – A Well-Fed World. awellfedworld.org/issues/animal protection

16. Food and Agriculture Organization of the U.N. FAOSTAT -Agriculture Livestock Primary Database, 2007. Chicken Meat, Slaughtered (Head). Available at:http:/faostat.fao.org/site/569/default.aspx#ancor.

17. Lourencetti C, Grimalt JO, Marco E, Fernandez P, Font-Ribera L, Villanueva CM, Kogevinas M: "Trihalomethanes in chlorine and bromine disinfected swimming pools: air-water distributions and human exposure." Environ Int. 45:59-67, Sep 15, 2012. EPub 2012 May 8.

18. Dioxin – Our Food –Database of Food and Related Sciences. 2012. www.ourfood.com/dioxin.html

19. National Cancer Institute http://www.cancer.gov/cancertopics/factsheet/Sites-Types/mesothelioma.

20. Wei B, Jia X, Ye B, Yu J, Zhang X, Lu R, Dong T, Yang L: "Impacts of land use on spatial distribution of mortality rates of cancers caused by naturally occurring asbestos." J. Exposure Science and Environmental Epidemiology 22 (5):516, Jul 4, 2012. Doi:10.1038/jes.2012.63.

21. http://consumerlawpage.com/article/fiber.shtml.

22. Karomi S, Boffetta P, Stewart PS, Brennan P, Zaridze D, Matveer V, Janout V, Kollarova H, Bencko V, Navratilova M, Szeszenia-Dabrowska N, Mates D, Gromiec J, Slamova A, Chow WH, Rothman N, Moore LE: "Occupational exposure to dusts and risk of renal cell carcinoma" Br. J. Cancer 104(11):1797-803, May 24, 2011. EPub 2011 May 3.

23. National Research Council: Biologic effects of ionizing radiation VII: Health risks from exposure to low levels of ionizing radiation. National Academy of Science, Washington D.C. 2005.

24. Boice JD: Radiation and breast carcinogenesis. Medical and Pediatric Oncology 36:508-513, 2001.

25. Harris S: "Organochlorine Contamination of Breast Milk" Environmental Defense Fund Nov. 7, 1979.

26. Regenstein L: How to Survive in America the Poisoned, Acropolis Books. P. 273, 1982.

Chapter 9 – Toxic Lifestyle Habits

1. Anad P, Kunnamakara AB, Sundaram C, Harikumar KB, Tharakan ST, Lai OS, Sung B, Aggarwal B: "Cancer is a Preventable Disease that Requires Major Lifestyle Changes." Pharmaceutical Research 25(9):2097-2116, Sep., 2008.

2. Campbell TC, Jacobson H: WHOLE. BenBella Books, Dallas, TX, 2013.

3. U.S. Department of Health and Human Services. The Health Consequences of Smoking: A Report of the Surgeon General. Atlanta: U.S. Department of Health and Human Services, Centers for Disease Control and Prevention, National Center for Chronic Disease Prevention and Health Promotion, Office on Smoking and Health, 2004.

4. Naimi T: Alcohol consumption is a leading preventable cause of cancer death in the U.S. American Journal of Public Health April, 2013. www.bumc.bu.edu/2013/alcohol.

5. Gu JW, Bailey AP, Sartin A, Makey I, Brady AL: Ethanol stimulates tumor progression and expression of vascular endothelial growth factor in chick embryos. Cancer 103(2):422-431, Jan 15, 2005.

6. Liu W, Swetzig WM, Medisetty R, Das GM: "Estrogen-mediated up regulation of NOXA is associated with cell cycle progression in estrogen receptor-positive breast cancer cells." PLoS 6(12): 2011.e29466. EPub Dec.22, 2011.

7. Xenoestrogen-wikipedia. en.wikipedia.org/wiki/xenoestogens

8. Ginat D: Xenoestrogens. www.alive.com/aricles/view/20q87 /xenoestrogens

9. Barton L: How to remove xenoestrogens. http://www.yahoo.com. eHow Contributor.

10. Karras T: Could Radiation Harm Your Health? Health P.92, July/August 2011.

11. Ben-Eliyahu S et al: "Stress Increases Metastatic Spread of a Mammary Tumor in Rats: Evidence for Mediation by the Immune System," Brain, Behavior, & Immunity 5(2):193-205, 1991.

12. Sapolsky RM, and Donnelly TM: "Vulnerability to Stress-Induced Tumor Growth Increases with Age in Rats: Role of Glucocorticoids," Endocrinology 117(2):662-66, 1985.

13. Thaker PH et al: "Chronic Stress Promotes Tumor Growth and Angiogenesis in a Mouse Model of Ovarian Carcinoma," Nature Medicine 12(8):939-44, 2006.

14. Servan-Schreiber D: Anticancer A New Way of Life. Penguin Group (USA) Inc., P. 152, 2009.

15. Consumer Reports on Health P.3, Jan 2012.

16. Sun Y, Campisi J, Higano C, Beer TM, Porter P, Coleman I, True L, Nelson PS: "Treatment-induced damage to the tumor microenvironment promotes prostate cancer therapy resistance through WNT16B." Nature Medicine 18(9):1359-68, Sept, 2012.

Chapter 10 – Toxic Diet

1. Israel B: How many cancers are caused by the environment? Scientific American May 21, 2010.

2. Nutritional Research Council. Diet, Nutrition, and Cancer. Washington: National Academy Press. 1982.

3. Obesity Worse for Health Than Drinking or Smoking. Public Health 115:229-235, 2001.

4. Beliveau R, Gingras D: Foods That Fight Cancer: Preventing Cancer Through Diet. New York: Random House. 2006.

5. Murray CJL, and Frenk J: Ranking 37th – Measuring the Performance of the U.S. Health Care System. N Engl J Med 362:98-99 Jan 14, 2010.

6. Food and Agriculture Organization of the U.N. FAOSTAT -Agriculture Livestock Primary Database, 2007. Chicken Meat, Slaughtered (Head). Available at:http:/faostat.fao.org/site/569/default.aspx#ancor.

7. Barnard ND: The Power of Your Plate. P.61. Book Publishing Company. 1990.

8. Armstrong B, Doll R: Environmental factors and cancer incidence and mortality in different countries, with special reference to dietary practices. International Journal of Cancer 15(4):617-31, 1975.

9. Campbell TC, Campbell II TM: The China Study. BenBella Books, Dallas, TX, 2005.

10. Nieves J, Cosman F, Herbert J et al: "High prevalence of vitamin D deficiency and reduced bone mass in multiple sclerosis." Neurology 44:1687-1692, 1994.

11. Chan JD, Stampfer MJ, Ma J et al: Insulin-like growth factor-1 (IGF-1) and IGF binding protein-3 as predictors of advanced-stage prostate cancer. Journal of National Cancer Institute 94(14):1099-106, Jul 17, 2002.

12. Inoue M, Iwasaki M, Otani T, Sasazuki S, Noda M, Tsugane S: Diabetes mellitus and the risk of cancer: results from a large-scale population-based cohort study in Japan. Archives of Internal Medicine 166(17):1871-1877, 2006.

13. Doi SQ, Rasaiah S, Tack I, Mysore J, Kopchick JJ, Moore J, Przemyslaw H, Striker JL, and Striker GE: Low-protein diet suppresses serum insulin-like growth factor-1 and decelerates the progression of growth hormone-induced glomerulosclerosis. Am J Nephrol. 21(4):331-339, Jul-Aug, 2001.

14. Allen NE, Appleby PN, Davey GK, Key TJ: Hormones and diet: low insulin-like growth factor-1 but normal bioavailable androgens in vegan men. Brit J Cancer 83(1):95-97, Jul, 2000.

15. Sood S: "Milking It, Why Monsanto Doesn't Want You to Know About Those Hormones in Your Dairy," Washington Independent. March 25, 2008.

16. Larsen HR: "Milk and the Cancer Connection," International Health News 76, April 1998. htpp://www.notmilk.com/drlarsen.html.

17. Colorectal (Colon) Cancer – Centers for Disease Control. www.cdc.gov/cancer/colorectal.

18. Schatzkin A, Park Y, Leitzmann MF et al: Prospective study of dietary fiber, whole grain foods, and small intestinal cancer. Gastroenterology 135(4):1163-1167, Oct 2008.

19. Park Y, Brinton LA, Subar AF, Hollenbeck A, Schatzkin A: Dietary fiber intake and risk of breast cancer in postmenopausal women: the National Institutes of Health-AARP Diet and Health Study. American J. Clinical Nutrition 90(3):664-71, Sep 2009.

20. Zheng W, Lee SA: "Well-done meat intake, heterocyclic amine exposure, and cancer risk. Nutri Cancer 61(4):437-46, 2009.

21. Liao GZ, Wang GY, Zhang YJ, Xu XL, Zhou GH: Formation of heterocyclic amines during cooking of duck meat. Food Addit Contam Part A Chem Anal Control Expo Risk Assess Jul 30, 2012. EPub ahead of print.

22. Jaret P: In Health P. 60, September/October, 1991.

23. Lauber SN, Gooderham NJ: The cooked meat-derived mammary carcinogen 2-amino-1-methyl-6-phenylimidazo [4, 5-b] pyridine promotes invasive behavior of breast cancer cells. Toxicology 279(1-3):139-145, 2011.

24. The Cancer Project Update: Cancer survivor sues over grilled chicken carcinogen. Good Medicine P.17, Winter 2010.

25. Reilly J: "Playing with Fire. Grilled chicken contains cancer-causing compounds." Good Medicine P.6-8, Summer, 2006.

26. Cho E, Chen WY, Hunter DJ, Stampfer MJ, Colditz GA, Hankinson SE, Willett WC: Red meat intake and risk of breast cancer among premenopausal women. Archive of Internal Medicine 166(20):2253-2259, 2006.

27. Hankinson SE, Willett WC, Colditz GA, Hunter DJ, Michaud DS, Deroo B, Rosner B, Speizer FE, Pollak M: Circulating concentration of insuln-like growth factor-1 and risk of breast cancer. The Lancet 351(9113):1393-1396, May 9, 1998.

28. Janssen J, and Lamberts S: Insulin-like growth factor-1 and risk of breast cancer. The Lancet 352:490, Aug. 8, 1998.

29. Norat T, Dossus L, Rinaldi S et al: Diet, serum insulin-like growth factor-1 and IGF-binding protein-3 in European women. European Journal of Clinical Nutrition 61(1):91-98, Jan 2007.

30. Goodson III WH: Milk products are a source of dietary progesterone. Abstract 202, San Antonio Breast Cancer Symposium December 2007. Available at:http://www.abstracts2view.com/sabcs/view.php/nu=SABCS07L-1108&terms=.

31. Hirayama T: Paper presented at Conference on Breast Cancer and Diet, U.S.-Japan Cooperative Cancer Research Program, Fred Hutchinson Cancer Center, Seattle, WA. March 14-15, 1977.

32. PCRM files lawsuit over carcinogens in grilled chicken. Good Medicine P.13, Winter 2007.

33. Vargas AJ, Thompson PA: Diet and nutrient factors in colorectal cancer risk. Nutr Clin Pract Aug 14, 2012. [Epub ahead of print].

34. Joshu CE, Parmigiani G, Colditz GA, Platz EA: Opportunities for the primary prevention of colorectal cancer in the United States. Cancer Prev Res (Phila) 5(1):138-45, Jan 2012.

35. Romaguera D, Vergnaud AC, Peeters P, van Gils CH, Chan DS et al: Is concordance with World Cancer Research Fund/American Institute for Cancer Research guidelines for cancer prevention related to subsequent risk of cancer? Results from the EPIC study. Am J Clin Nutr 96(1):150-63, Jul 2012.

36. Perez-Cueto FJ, Verbeke W: Consumer implications of the WCRF's permanent update on colorectal cancer. Meat Science 90(4):977-8, Apr 2012.

37. World Cancer Research Fund/American Institute for Cancer Research. Food, Nutrition, Physical Activity, and the Prevention of Cancer: A Global Perspective. Washington, DC:AICR, 2007.

38. Larsson SC, Orsini N, Wolk A: Processed meat consumption and stomach cancer risk: a meta-analysis. Journal of National Cancer Institute 98 (15):1078-1087, Aug 2, 2006.

39. Robbins J: "Meat-Packer Defends Beef." Riverside Herald, May 8, 1976. Diet for a New America. Stillpoint Publishing. 1987.

40. Zhang J, Zhao Z, Berkel HJ: Egg consumption and mortality from colon and rectal cancers: an ecological study. Nutrition Cancer 46(2):158-165, 2003.

41. Iscovich JM, L'Abbe KA, Castelleto R: Colon Cancer in Argentina. I: Risk from intake of dietary items. II: Risk from fibre, fat and nutrients. International Journal of Cancer 51(6):851-861, 1992.

42. Integrative Medicine: a Clinician's Journal P. 50, June/July 2007.

43. Phillips R: "Role of Lifestyle and Dietary Habits in Risk of Cancer" Cancer Research 35:3513-22, 1975.

44. Richman EL, Kenfield SA, Stampfer MJ, Giovannucci EL, Chan JM: Egg, red meat, and poultry intake and risk of lethal prostate cancer in the prostate specific antigen-era: incidence and survival. Cancer Prev Res 4(12):2110-21, Dec 2011.

45. Tate PL, Bibb R, Larcom, LL: "Milk stimulates growth of prostate cancer cells in culture." Nutrition Cancer 63(8):1361-6, Nov, 2011. EPub 2011 Nov 1.

46. Bravi F, Scotti L, Bosetti C et al: Self-reported history of hypercholesterolemia and gallstones and the risk of prostate cancer. Annuals of Oncology 17(6):1014-1017, June 2006.

47. Glade MJ: Food, nutrition, and the prevention of cancer: a global perspective. American Institute for Cancer Research/World Cancer Research Fund, American Institute for Cancer Research. 1997. Nutrition 15(6):523-6, June 1999.

48. Chan JM, Stampfer MJ, Ma J, Gann PH, Gasiano JM, Giovannucci E: Dairy products, calcium, and prostate cancer risk in the Physicians' Health Study. Am J Clinical Nutrition 74(4):549-54, Oct 2001.

49. Tseng MM, Breslow RA, Graubard BI, Ziegler RG: Dairy, calcium and vitamin D intakes and prostate cancer risk in the National Health and Nutrition Examination Epidemiologic Follow-up Study cohort. Am J Clinical Nutrition 81(5):1147-54, May 2005.

50. Kats AE: "The Holistic Approach to Prostate Health." Integrative Medicine 6(3):57, June/July 2007.

51. Kiani F, Knutsen S, Singh P, Ursin G, Fraser G: Dietary risk factors for ovarian cancer: the Adventist Health Study United States. Cancer Causes Control 17(2):137-46, Mar 2006.

52. Zhang M, Yang Z.Y, Binns CW, Lee AH: Diet and ovarian cancer risk: a case-control study in China. Br. J of Cancer 86(5):712-7, Mar 4, 2002.

53. Kushi LH, Mink PL, Folsom AR, Anderson K.E, Zheng W, Lazovich D, Sellers TA: Prospective study of diet and ovarian cancer. Am J Epidemiology 149(1):21-31, Jan 1999.

54. Larsson SC, Bergkvist, L, Wolk A: Milk and lactose intakes and ovarian cancer risk in the Swedish Mammography Cohort. Am J Clinical Nutrition 80(5):1353-7, Nov 2004.

55. Cramer DW, Harlow BL, Willett WC, Welch WR, Bell DA, Scully RE, Ng WG, Knapp RC: Galactose consumption and metabolism in relation to the risk of ovarian cancer. Lancet 2(8654):66-71, Jul 8, 1989.

56. King MG, Olson SH, Paddock L, Chasdran V, Demissie K, Lu SE, Parekh N, Rodriguez-Rodriguez L, Bandera EV: Sugary food and beverage consumption and epithelial ovarian cancer risk: a population-based case-control study. BMC Cancer 13:94; Feb 27, 2013.

57. Mills PK, Beeson WL, Abbey DE, Fraser GE, Phillips RL: Dietary habits and past medical history as related to fatal pancreas cancer risk among Adventists. Cancer 61(12):2578-85, Jun 15, 1988.

58. Larsson SC, Wolk A: Red and processed meat consumption and risk of pancreatic cancer: meta-analysis of prospective studies. British Journal of Cancer 106(3):603-7, Jan 31, 2012.

59. "Sour News About Sweet Drinks" American Heart Association's Scientific Sessions, 2011. Natural Awakenings P.11, May 2012.

60. Grothey A, Voigt C, Schober C, Muller T, Dempke W, Schmoll HJ: The role of insulin-like growth factor I and its receptor in cell growth, transformation, apoptosis, and chemoresistance in solid tumors. Journal Cancer Research & Clinical Oncology 125(3-4):166-73, 1999.

61. Long L, Navab R, Brod P: Regulation of the Mr 72,000 type IV collagenase by the type 1 insulin-like growth factor receptor. Cancer Research 58(15):3243-47, Aug 1, 1998.

62. Moeller SM, Fryhofer SA, Osbahr III AJ, Robinowitz CB: The effects of high fructose syrup. Journal of American College of Nutrition 28(6):619-26, Dec 2009.

63. Weil A: Is High-Fructose Corn Syrup Bad for You? Health.Com P.20, October 2010.

64. Wallace R: Don't be Fooled by "Corn Sugar". Tasteforlife P.24, September 2011.

65. Beware of high-fructose corn syrup. Consumer Reports on Health p.2, March 2013.

66. Jee SH, Ohrr H, Sull JW, Yun JE, Ji M, Samet JM: Fasting serum glucose level and cancer risk in Korean men and women, JAMA 293(2):194-202, Jan 12, 2005.

67. Hoehn SK, Carrol KK: Effects of dietary carbohydrate on the incidence of mammary tumors induced in rats by 7,12-dimethylbenz-anthracene. Nutrition and Cancer 1(3):27-30, 1979.

68. Olney JW, Farber NB, Spitznagel E, Robins LN: Increasing brain tumor rates: is there a link to aspartame? J of Neuropathology and Experimental Neurology 55(11):1115-23, Nov 1996.

69. Blaylock R: Excitotoxins -The Taste that Kills. Health Press. P.21, 1994.

70. Desmeules M, Mikkelsen T, Mao Y: Increasing incidence of primary malignant brain tumors: Influence of diagnostic methods." Journal of National Cancer Institute 84(6):442-445, Mar 18, 1992.

71. Levy PS, Hedeker D: Statistical and epidemiological treatment of the SEER incidence data. J of Neuropathology and Experimental Neurology 55(12):1280, Dec 1996.

72. Roberts HJ: "Does Aspartame Cause Human Brain Cancer," Journal of Advancement in Medicine 4 (4):231-41, 1991.

73. Soffritti M, Belpoggi F, Degli ED, Lambertin L, Tibald E, Rigano A: First experimental demonstration of the multipotential carcinogenic effects of aspartame administered in the feed to Sprague-Dawley rats, Environmental Health Perspectives 114(3):379-85, Mar 2006.

74. AARP The Magazine P.14, 2006.

75. Li J, Thompson TD, Miller JW, Pollack LA, Stewart SL: Cancer incidence among children and adolescents in the United States, 2001-2003. Pediatrics 121(6):e1470-7, Jun; 2008. Doi:10.1542/ped.2007-2974.

76. 'Feel-good' food might be addictive. Consumer Reports on Health November 2012 p.10.

77. Time P.20, June 18, 2012.

78. Horne S: Protecting yourself from xenoestrogens. http//www.naturalnutritionresource.

79. Fuhrman J: Eat to Live. Little, Brown and Company. 2011.

80. Walker N: The Natural Way to Vibrant Health Norwalk Press. 1972.

81. Young MR, Young ME: Effects of fish oil and corn oil diets on prostaglandin-dependent and myelopoiesis-associated immune suppressor mechanisms of mice bearing metastatic Lewis lung carcinoma tumors. Cancer Research 49(8):1931-6, April 15, 1989.

82. Coulombe J, Pelletier G, Tremblay P, Mercier G, Oth D: Influence of lipid diets on the number of metastases and ganglioside content of H59 variant tumors. Clin Exp Metastasis 15(4):410-7, July 1997.

83. Turner L: Oil Change. Vegetarian Times P.66, Nov 2011.

84. Barnard ND: The Edge Against Cancer. Vegetarian Times P.18, October 1991.

85. Harris RB, Foote JA, Hakim IA, Bronson DL, Alberts DS: Fatty acid composition of red blood cell membranes and risk of squamous cell carcinoma of the skin. Cancer Epidemiology Biomarkers Prev. 14(4):906-12, April 2005.

86. Harper HA, Rodwell VW, Mayes PA: Review of physiological chemistry 16th edition. Lange Medical Publications. 1977.

87. Ornish D: Dr. Dean Ornish's Program for Reversing Heart Disease. Random House Inc., 1990.

88. Anderson M: Healing Cancer from Inside Out. 2009. www.RaveDiet.com.

89. Warburg O: The Prime Cause and Prevention of Cancer. The meeting of the Nobel-Laureates. June 30, 1966.

90. Sidney S, Farquhar JW: Cholesterol, cancer, and public health policy. Am J Med. 75(3):494-508, Sep 1983.

91. Cruse JP: Dietary cholesterol deprivation improves survival and reduces incidence of metastatic colon cancer in dimethylhydrazine-pretreated rats. Gut. 23(7):594-9, Jul 1982.

92. Chen HW, Kandutsch AA, Heiniger HJ: The role of cholesterol in malignancy. Prog Exp Tumor Res. 22:275-316, 1978.

93. Mady EA: Association between estradiol, estrogen receptors, total lipids, triglycerides, and cholesterol in patients with benign and malignant breast tumors. J Steroid Biochem Mol Biol. 75(4-5):323-8, Dec 31, 2000.

94. Ireland C: Hormones in milk can be dangerous. Harvard University Gazette. Dec. 7, 2006.

95. Farlow D W, Xu X, Veenstra TD: Quantitative measurement of endogenous estrogen metabolites, risk- factors for development of breast cancer, in commercial milk products by LC-MS/MS. J Chromto B. 877(13).1327-1334. May, 2009.

Chapter 11 – My Nutrition Research

1. Cook BB, Lau EW, Bailey BM: The Protein Quality of Waste-grown Green Algae. I. Quality of protein mixtures of algae, nonfat powdered milk, and cereals. Journal of Nutrition 81:23-29, 1963.

2. Campbell TC and Campbell II TM: The China Study. BenBella Books, Dallas, TX, P.104, 2005.

3. Kirschner H, E: Live Food Juices. H. E. Kirschner Publications. P. 93, 1991.

Chapter 12 – Phytotherapy – Crux of the Matter

1. Food, Nutrition & Herbs! Phytochemicals.
   www.bellybytes.com /phytochemicals.

2. Fuhrman J: Super Immunity. Health.com October 2011.

3. Barrie L: These Foods Fight Cancer. Health P.113, November 2010.

4. www.cancer.org/phytochemicals.

5. Kushi LH, Doyle C, McClullough M et al: American Cancer Society guidelines on nutrition and physical activity for cancer prevention: Reducing the risk of cancer with healthy food choices and physical activity. CA Cancer J Clin. 62(1):30-67; 2012.

6. Zhang CX, Ho SC, Chen YM, Fu JH, Cheng SZ, Lin FY: "Greater vegetable and fruit intake is associated with a lower risk of breast cancer among Chinese women." Int. J Cancer 125(1):181-8, Jul 1, 2009.

7. Iscovich JM, L'Abbe KA, Castelleto R: Colon cancer in Argentina II: Risk from fibre, fat and nutrients. International J of Cancer 51(6):858-61, 1992.

Chapter 13 – The Reverse Diet

1. Kirschner HE: Live Food Juices. H. E. Kirschner Publications. P. 20, 1991.
2. Walker NW: Fresh Vegetable and Fruit Juices. Norwalk Press P.19, 1970.
3. Quigley D: 10 Benefits and Uses for Miso. Care 2 Healthy Living. www.Care 2.com.
4. Kessman S: The Health Benefits of Miso Soup: Japanese Chicken Soup. May 16, 2006.
5. Keough J: "A Killer Kitchen Spice" Alternative Medicine P. 25, September 2006.

Chapter 14 – The Recovery Diet

1. Ornish D, Lin J, Chan JM, et al: Effect of comprehensive lifestyle changes on telomerase activity and telomere length in men with biopsy-proven low-risk prostate cancer: 5-year follow-up of a descriptive pilot study. Lancet Oncol. 17 September 2013. DOI:10.1016/S1470-2045(13)70366-8.
2. NEWSTART is a registered trademark of Weimar Center, 20601 W. Paoli Lane, P.O. Box 486, Weimar, CA 95736.
3. Wikipedia.org/wiki/Battle_Creek_Sanitarium
4. Davies NJ, Batchup L, Thomas R: The role of diet and physical activity in breast, colorectal, and prostate cancer survivorship: a review of the literature. Br J Cancer 105 suppl 1:s52-73, Nov 8, 2011.
5. Water. Amazing Health Facts! Amazing Facts, Inc. 2009.
6. Altieri A, La Vecchia C, Negri E: Fluid intake and risk of bladder and other cancers. European J of Clinical Nutrition 57, suppl 2:s59-s68, 2003. Doi:10, 1038/sj.ejen.1601903.
7. Lau BH: Hydrotherapy for Flu and Respiratory Infections. 2010.
8. Adams M: Natural Health Solutions. Incubation Books, Ventura, CA, P.302, 2006.
9. Robsahm T, Tretli S, Dahlback A, Moan J: Vitamin D3 from sunlight may improve the prognosis of breast-, colon- and prostate cancer (Norway). Cancer Causes Control (2):149-58, March 2004.
10. Grant W: Reduce your risk of cancer with sunlight exposure. Mercola.com. March 31, 2004.
11. Garland C, Garland F, Gorham E, Lipkin M, Newmark H, Mohr S, Holick M: The Role of Vitamin D in Cancer Prevention. American Journal of Public Health 96(2) 252-261, February, 2006.
12. Pierre C: "The Sunshine Vitamin Are You Getting Enough?" AARP. P. 18, September & October, 2009.
13. Matilda B: Lack of sleep dramatically alters genes. Science World Report. Feb. 2013. Scienceworldreport.com/..of sleep_ alters_genes.

14. St. Lifer, H: Fight Back Against Breast Cancer. AARP. P. 16, October & November, 2013.

15. P53 Gene. Wikipedia.org.

16. Newberg AB, Waldman MR: Why We Believe What We Believe: Our Biological Need for Meaning, Spirituality, and Truth. Free Press. 2006.

Chapter 15 – The Right Diet

1. Santillo H: Food Enzymes The Missing Link to Radiant Health.1991.

2. Klatz R, and Goldman R: 7 Anti-Aging Secrets for Optimal Digestion and Scientific Weight Loss. Elite Sports Medicine Publications. P 32, 1996.

3. Singh SV, Warin R, Xia D et al: Sulforaphane inhibits prostate carcinogenesis and pulmonary metastasis in TRAMP mice in association with increased cytotoxicity of natural killer cells. Cancer Research 69(5):2117-25, Mar 1, 2009.

4. Moiseeva EP, Heukers R, Manson MM: EGFR and Src are involved in indole-3-carbinol-induced death and cell cycle arrest of human breast cancer cells. Carcinogenesis 28(2):435-45, Feb 2007.

5. Broccoli compound helps destroy breast cancer cells. Good Medicine P. 17, Spring 2007.

6. Do R, Xie C, Zhang X, Mannisto S, Harald K, Islam S et al: The effect of chromosome 9p21 viariants on cardiovascular disease may be modified by dietaryintake:evidence from a case/control and a prospective study. PLoS Medicine 8(10):e1001106, Oct.11, 2011.

7. P53 Gene. Wikipedia.org.

8. Mirzayans R, Andrais B, Scott A, Murray D: New insights into p53 signaling and cancer cell response to DNA damage: implications for cancer therapy. J. Biomed Biotechnol. 2012:170325. Epub 2012 Jul15.

9. Rogers SA: The Cholesterol Hoax. Sand Key Company, Inc. Sarasota, FL, P. 177, 367, 374, 2008.

10. Tallmadge K: "How Healthy Is Your Favorite Veggie?" Vegetarian Times P.27-28, April 2005.

11. Barrie L: These Foods fight Cancer. Health P.113, November, 2010.

12. Seeram NP, Aviram M, Zhang Y, Henning SM, Feng L, Dreher M, Herber D: Comparison of antioxidant potency of commonly consumed polyphenol-rich beverages in the United States. J Agric Food Chem. 56(4):1415-22, Feb 27, 2008.

13. Pomegranate Juice Fights Lung Cancer, Prostate Cancer, Colon Cancer and Breast Cancer. May 15, 2010.

14. www.jmbblog.com/2010/05/.64-pomegranate-juice-and-extracts.

15. Pantuck AJ, Leppert JT, Zomorodian N et al: Phase II study of pomegranate juice for men with rising prostate-specific antigen following surgery or radiation for prostate cancer. Clinical Cancer Research 12(13):4018-26, Jul 1, 2006.

16. Troll W, Wiesner R, Shellabarger C J, Holtzman S, Stone JP: "Soybean diet lowers breast tumor incidence in irradiated rats." Carcinogenesis (6):4691-72 Jun 1980.
17. Zaizen Y, Higuchi Y, Matsuo N, Shirabe K, Tokuda H, Takeshita M: Antitumor effects of soybean hypocotyls and soybeans on the mammary tumor induction by N-methyl-n-nitrosourea in F344 rats. Anticancer Res. 20(3A):1439-44, May-Jun, 2000.
18. Cronkite C: The Top Ten Anti-Cancer Causing Foods. May 11, 2011. www.livestrong.com/article/438994-the-top-ten-anti...
19. Galloway L: "How peppers can fire up your health." Naturalsolutionsmag.com.
20. Jagetia GC, Aggarwal BB: "Spicing Up" of the immune system by curcumin. Journal of Clinical Immunology 27(1):19-35, Jan 2007.
21. Aune D, Chan D, Lau R et al: Dietary fibre, whole grains, and risk of colorectal cancer: systematic review and dose-response meta-analysis of prospective studies. BMJ 343:d6617, Nov 10, 2011.
22. Aubertin-Leheudre M, Hamalainen E, Adlercreutz H: Diets and hormonal levels in postmenopausal women with or without breast cancer. Nutr Cancer 63(4):514-524, 2011.
23. Gonzales J, Levin S: Vegetarian Diets Help Expel Cancer-Causing Hormones. Good Medicine P.17, Winter 2012.
24. Puotinen CJ: "Green Superfoods for Numerous Benefits." Taste for Life P. 44, April, 2009.

Chapter 16 – Why Buy Organic?

1. Sustainable Food News. July, 2011.
2. Hsu-LeBlanc E: "Buy Organic." Taste for Life April, 2009.
3. Fitzgerald R: "Organic Food, A Consumer Scam?" Healing Our World. Hippocrates Health Institute. 29(36), 2010.
4. Ambrose E: "How to Eat Organically Without Going Broke." Buy Organic P. 12, 2011
5. http://www.fruitsticker.com.
6. Reistad-Long S: "11 Things It's Best to Buy Organic." Health P.133, April, 2011.
7. Edwards K: "Eat Clean for Less -The New Dirty Dozen." Vegetarian Times P. 74-77, September 2011.

Index

204, 219, 252, 274–275, 283

B

baby Bella mushrooms 274
bacillus Calmette-Guerin 19
bacteria 45–46, 48–49, 51
balsamic vinegar 186, 208, 218, 239–240
banana 109, 145, 155–156, 164, 167, 180, 283, 295
barley flour 165
barley grass 140, 155
basil 137, 170, 203, 213, 223, 227, 232, 263, 265–267
B cells 47–48, 50
BCG 19
bean sprouts 252
beet 18, 116, 118–119, 137, 155, 157, 159, 237–238
Beijing Cancer Hospital 25
bell peppers 116, 137, 145, 157, 169, 177, 182, 185–186, 190, 193, 224–225, 233, 235–236, 250, 252–254, 256–257, 265, 270, 299
berries 10, 137, 139, 143
beverages 51
BIG FAVOR 111, 141
Bill's Baste and Marinade 220
Bill's Chik'nish 222
bioflavonoids 30, 138
black beans 138, 165, 173, 177, 189, 219–220, 243
bladder cancer 18–20, 24, 66, 70, 124, 200
blindfolding 8, 16, 24
blueberries 137, 140, 145, 185, 257
blue-green algae 155
B lymphocyte 47, 51–52
BPA 72
Bragg Liquid Aminos 171–172, 181, 186, 190, 194–196, 203, 205–206, 208, 212–213, 216, 218, 227, 229, 231, 233, 235,

237, 239–240, 242–243, 246, 249–250, 254, 256, 258–261, 263–265, 268, 297–298, 300, 307
brain 51
brain cancer 18, 37, 72, 91, 329
breads and crackers 276
breakfast recipes 161
breast cancer xiii, 1–3, 21, 27–28, 37, 40–41, 49–50, 54, 56, 61–62, 64, 69–70, 77, 84–86, 94, 108–109, 117, 124–126, 138–139, 180, 191, 212, 220, 245, 252, 260, 269, 274–275, 293, 301, 304, 313, 316, 319, 321, 324–326, 330, 332–333
Breast Carcinoma Associated Antigen 27.29 64
Brenda Cobb 55
Brian Clement 58
Brian Wong ix, 23–24, 26
broccoli 10, 18, 107, 116, 136–137, 158, 177, 179–180, 332
brown rice 129, 133–134, 220, 243–245, 248–250, 267, 290
Brussels sprouts 18, 136–137, 203–204, 218
Burkitt's lymphoma 23
butternut squash 169, 174, 226, 270–271
button mushrooms 140, 171, 203, 212, 227, 250

C

CA 15-3 64
cabbage 10, 18, 116, 136, 145, 158, 172, 178, 186, 214–215, 218, 226, 241, 254–255, 257
caffeine 48, 50, 109, 134, 284, 286
Caldwell B. Esselstyn 3
cancer 46, 48, 52
cancer cells 48
Cancer Project 1, 313, 318, 326
cancers 49

gluten 102, 172, 216, 226, 231, 249–250, 255, 298
grapefruit 137, 145
grape-nut cereal 291
grapes 51, 137, 145, 190, 257, 291, 293
green apple 158, 182
green onions 181–182, 185–186, 189, 213–214, 219, 224, 233, 235, 242, 252, 254, 258–259
green powder 103, 114–115, 129, 132, 155–156
green tea 134, 140

H

Hallelujah Acres 68–69, 309, 321
Hannah Wong 24
hay fever 52
heart 51
heart disease 2–4, 33, 35–36, 48, 51, 83, 108, 136, 156, 171, 173, 176, 180, 185, 189, 191, 199, 217, 221–222, 230, 243, 249, 253, 257, 277, 280, 283, 287, 289, 306, 313, 318, 320, 329
heliotherapy 63, 124
hemp protein 156
hemp seeds 162–163, 192, 293, 307
Hepatitis B and C viruses 23
herbal formula 25, 27–28
Herbert C. Ruckle 19
Hodgkin's disease 53–54
Holy Bible 148
homemade almond butter 296, 306
homemade soy yogurt 195, 296, 302
Human Papilloma virus 23
hydrotherapy 42, 63–64, 66, 124, 331

I

IgE antibodies 52
immune cells xi, xii, 8–10, 24, 48–51, 58–59, 62, 70, 89, 106–108, 122, 137, 147, 149, 204
immune system xi, 4, 7, 10, 19, 46–52,
58–59, 63, 73, 75, 77, 79–80, 89, 93–95, 105–106, 123, 131, 140, 148, 155, 157, 160, 163, 173, 195, 198, 215, 221, 229, 238–239, 245, 247, 271, 319–321, 324, 333
immunotherapy xi, 7, 19–20, 25, 70, 147, 313–314, 316
infections 47, 49
influenza 45
initiation 8, 22
innate immunity 45
insulin-like growth factor 83–84, 90, 94, 325–326, 328
interferons 46, 239
in vitro model 20–21, 24–25, 316

J

jalapeno peppers 193
James L. Woolley 19
James M. Slater 11, 14
Jeffrey Tosk 20
Jerry R. Rittenhouse 24
Joel Fuhrman 107
John Harvey Kellogg 122
John McDougall 4
Journal of Urology 20, 24, 41, 313–314, 316–318
juicer xiii, 116, 157–160, 306

K

kale 10, 18, 116, 136–137, 143, 145, 155, 157–158, 160, 177, 179–180, 186, 204, 228, 252, 296, 307
kamut 190–191
Karolinska Institute 39
kelp 203, 216, 226, 252, 268–269, 298
ketchup 94, 102, 195, 220, 233, 249, 263
kidney beans 177, 185, 188, 197, 257, 290
kidney cancer 24–26, 70
kiwi 145

www.ingramcontent.com/pod-product-compliance
Lightning Source LLC
Chambersburg PA
CBHW020725180526
45163CB00001B/107